"An informative, easy-to-read, engaging and understandable book about living with a low grade brain tumour, peppered with a range of real-life experiences from different people as well as Gideon's own story. Highly recommended for those living with a low grade brain tumour, but also other brain tumour patients, carers, family and friends to help understand what a loved one is going through and the journey ahead."
Sarah Lindsell, Chief Executive
The Brain Tumour Charity

"For too long low grades have been the Cinderella of brain tumours. Not any more. For the first time these quietly dangerous tumours have been put under the spotlight. With real understanding, Gideon captures the very wearing toll that living with a low grade tumour creates. But he counters it with humour and optimism without compromising honesty. This book is a must-read for anyone living with a low grade brain tumour as a patient, carer or friend."
Helen Bulbeck, Director
brainstrust

"This book is an important addition to the increasing library of works being published by outstanding individuals living with brain tumours and impassioned to do something to help others. We congratulate Gideon on his efforts and would encourage anyone diagnosed with a low grade brain tumour to read this valuable account of his experiences."
Sue Farrington Smith, Chief Executive
Brain Tumour Research

First published in Great Britain in 2013
by ngo.media limited

Brain Tumours: Living low grade

A catalogue record for this book is available
from the British Library.

Paperback ISBN: 978-0-9553695-7-5
Also available on Kindle

Published by ngo.media limited
Austons, Layer Road, Abberton CO5 7NH
Company registration number: 04916846

2 4 6 8 10 9 7 5 3 1

Cover design: Chandler Book Design
www.chandlerbookdesign.co.uk

Printed by CreateSpace

Brain Tumours
Living low grade

The patient guide to life with
a slow growing brain tumour

GIDEON BURROWS

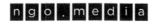

For the patients who told me their stories and for Richard who
met me at a train station and made me feel better

Gideon Burrows was diagnosed with an incurable inoperable low
grade glioma brain tumour aged 35. He is a writer, small business
owner and involved father. He lives close to the sea in Essex, owns
five bicycles and grows 13 varieties of chillies

www.bicyclesandbraintumours.co.uk

Contents

Introduction

"THE BETTER END of the bad ones."

That's how I got used to describing my brain tumour to friends and family, to somehow explain why I happened to be still alive.

That was a few months in, after the initial shock. And after I'd found out a little more for myself about low grade glioma brain tumours.

My wife and I had been told in a hospital corridor that I had a Grade II tumour, probably a glioma. There and then the surgeon had said I wasn't going to die just yet.

"These tumours are measured in years, not months," he'd said. "Sometimes many, many years."

But I wasn't listening. All I'd heard were the words 'brain' and 'tumour' and 'die'. Nothing else mattered.

After all, a brain tumour is a brain tumour right? The worst of the worst. A death sentence.

So it was with not a little surprise that we left the hospital with just a one-page poorly-photocopied leaflet on brain tumours, a prescription for epilepsy drugs and advice from a nurse to not go Googling my condition. Something I of course

1

did as soon as I got home.

After dropping such a bombshell, the consultant had said I should simply go away and get on with my life. Come back in three months for another MRI scan and we'll check in to see how things are going.

That, I now know, is what living low grade is all about. Life in three- six- or 12-month chunks, not quite knowing what even the near future will bring.

This book is for the hundreds of people, as well as their families and friends, who are diagnosed in the UK every year with a low grade glioma. Gliomas are by far the most common form of brain tumour. And a low grade one (Grades I and II) is not always benign, but nor is it – or at least not yet – a malignant cancer.

That little leaflet I was handed at the hospital on diagnosis day contained very little about low grade brain tumours. A couple of lines at most. It was surrounded by paragraphs about life-threatening childhood brain cancer and information on higher grade brain tumours (Grades III and IV). The latter had life expectancy that *was* measured in a few months, sometimes just a year or two.

It was a pattern I found repeated across other information sources: websites, cancer charities, in consultants' clinics and in media stories. Information was rich for immediately life-threatening brain tumours, but very scarce on long-term versions like low grade gliomas.

It was the Cinderella of brain cancer. Left to get on with it at home, while the more *serious* brain tumours got all the bright lights and attention.

Of course there was technical information if you looked for it. About types and research, as well as about treatments. But there was next to nothing about trying to live your life with a low grade glioma. There was little about the changes in your day-to-day existence, the emotional impact, the uncertainty, the treatments and drugs, the limbo, the guilt of having one of the 'better end of the bad ones'. The fear that for many of us our tumours *will* eventually end our lives.

I hope this book fills the gap. It follows my own story of how my Grade II glioma was discovered and its progress. I share what low grade gliomas are and how they work. And how I learned – the hard way, because no-one really ever explained it – to get used to living with one.

With brain tumours, everyone's experience is different. This book also features the experiences of other low grade tumour patients and those of their families. I share the stories of over 20 patients who have been generous with their time and honest with their contributions. Some testimonies come from brain tumour patients whose low grade tumours are not gliomas, but whose experiences are likely to resonate. This book simply would not have happened without everyone who was kind enough to tell their story.

You'll also find non-technical information about tumour types, treatments and options. But this is a layperson's book, not a scientific manual.

There are over 900 people diagnosed with a low grade glioma every year in the UK. For some of us, doctors will want to move to surgery straight away. For others, early radiotherapy or chemotherapy might be the preferred option. For some it'll be a combination of all these things. For still more – as it was for me – consultants will initially advocate a watch and wait policy.

Our journeys might vary, but most of us will be united by a common thread. A sometimes life-limiting illness, but one that is long drawn out. Difficult to deal with month after month, year after year. We spend most days of our lives acutely conscious that we have a brain tumour. Many of us will experience frequent and serious side effects like seizures, nausea, memory loss, physical weakness, sight problems and disability. We may be banned from driving, from drinking alcohol and have a daily drug regime to keep everything at bay. Yet, many of us are also expected to carry on with our lives as if very little has changed.

Some of the things I've written will resonate with you and some will help. Some will do neither. That's the nature of such a diverse disease. The location of the tumour in the brain, its type and even its genetic makeup can offer radically different outcomes and treatment options from patient to patient.

This book is primarily aimed at adults who have been diagnosed with a low grade glioma. Average age of diagnosis is between 30- and 50-years-old. In fact, it has struck me particularly hard while working on this book how many of those who have contributed are younger than my own tender 36 years.

But I do hope it will also help parents of children with a low grade diagnosis. In the book there are two mothers whose children are on their own brain tumour journeys. They share their own experiences.

Together, we and our families are all living low grade. Though it sometimes doesn't feel like it, our experiences, our feelings, our lives are just as important and complex as those with more immediately malignant brain tumours. I hope this little book helps fill a large gap that has been left open for too long.

Gideon Burrows
36, oligodendroglioma Grade II

What this book isn't

This isn't a technical book. There's information out there already about medical terms, specific names for specific cells, and the intricacies of how treatments and brain illnesses operate. Instead of repeating that material, I aim to offer the human, emotional and practical side to living with a low grade brain tumour.

I include technical information only where necessary. And then only in brief. Hopefully I'll provide enough information for you to ask your own questions and do your own research about the more technical side of things. Doctors and nurses may urge us not to go searching on Google, but can they blame us when the information provided can sometimes be so lacking?

This book also isn't about dying. It's about living and coping with a low grade brain tumour, a tumour that is life-limiting in many cases but not yet life-threatening.

I briefly cover transformation from low grade tumours to higher grade ones, and in a very general way preparing for the longer-term implications. But there isn't the space or intention here to include detailed information about higher grade brain gliomas, nor specific information about what might happen when low grades turn malignant.

I focus specifically on the difficulties and adaptations we low graders have to make after diagnosis, and then in living with our brain tumours day-to-day. That's enough to cope with in itself.

The resources section aims to help you widen your knowledge and to begin to gather more detailed information about your own condition.

1

In it for the long haul

LET'S GET ONE thing straight before we start. If you have just been diagnosed with a low grade glioma, you're very unlikely to die any time soon.

Despite assuming – as I did – that a brain tumour was an immediate death sentence, I'm still very much alive, pretty healthy and that's unlikely to change in the near future. Gliomas may be the most common type of brain tumour, making up half of all primary brain tumours, but having the low grade version is far more rare than having a high grade one. And even though low grade gliomas are far less common than higher grades, they have a far longer life expectancy. As one talk board contributor put it:

> "The only reality is that my wife and I know that she is not likely to live to old age and that whatever finally gets her, it is more likely to be the tumour than anything else."

In a sense, we're the lucky ones. It is hard to listen when we're first diagnosed, but being told we have a low grade glioma really is to have 'the better end of the bad ones'.

Let's get the basic medical stuff out of the way first, before we get on to living with a low grade glioma.

Low grade what...?

To keep things neat and tidy for medical establishments the world over, the World Health Organization (WHO) has introduced a classification system for brain tumours. They're identified by examining cells from the tumour under a microscope. Low grades are I and II; high grades are III and IV. The higher grade your tumour, the more abnormal the cells inside the tumour are and the more malignant it is. Most low grade gliomas are Grade II brain tumours, though there are a few Grade I versions too.

Grade I glioma tumours mostly occur in children, though they do occur in adults too. They rarely progress to a higher grade, so aren't considered life-threatening unless they are in a dangerous position. Though they certainly can have life-changing effects.

Grade II tumours more frequently occur in adults, and they do have the potential to transform into Grade III or IV tumours. Their rate of growth and transformation, though unpredictable, tends to be slow.

Non-childhood low grade gliomas usually occur in people in their 30s and 40s, malignant Grade III and IV gliomas occur at any time in a person's life, but are most common among people in their 50s and 60s.

Gliomas are a type of brain tumour that emerges from the glial cells in the brain. Glial cells are not responsible for the thinking, processing, 'braininess' of our brain. Rather unglamorously, they're more like the glue that holds those cells together and protects them.

In very broad terms, a glioma brain tumour occurs when one of those cells goes wrong and starts multiplying uncontrollably. But these glial brain cells can also be subdivided into different types, all doing subtly different things. That's what creates the different types of gliomas. In fact, there are subtypes even of those different types, but let's keep things relatively simple.

What's important to remember is that while doctors can often tell you exactly what kind of low grade glioma you have after a biopsy or surgery, impact and prognosis is bound to vary from person to person. That's because tumours vary in size, growth rates, location and aggressiveness.

It is worth going over the basic types of low grade glioma, so we know where we stand.

Astrocytoma

These Grade II tumours are the most common form of low grade glioma. We often assume tumours to be like a solid lump, but gliomas including the astrocytoma tend to be more diffuse. Imagine a coral like shape, with tentacles reaching out and infusing into the healthy tissue. Astrocytomas are usually diagnosed in patients in their late 30s.

Pilocytic astrocytoma

These are Grade I tumours, almost exclusively diagnosed in children and young adults. They tend to be very slow growing indeed, and many can be cured by surgery.

Oligodendroglioma

A slow growing Grade II tumour that grows out of the fatty sheath that covers and protects brain cells. Imagine the white plastic covering of the wires into a plug and you get a general idea of what cells oligodendrogliomas emerge from.

Ganglioglioma

These are slow growing low grade tumours, actually emerging from both glial cells and ganglion cells (which are brain cells proper). They're usually benign, though in some cases can transform into higher grade tumours.

Mixed glioma

Some gliomas can be a mix of the subtypes: astrocytoma and oligodendroglioma. This type of tumour is also known as an oligo-astrocytoma or astro-oligodendroglioma, depending on which originating cell is dominant. They also tend to be treated according to whichever element is dominant.

Ependymoma

These are the rarest type of low grade glioma. They mostly occur in children and are mostly Grade I. However they can progress to Grade III, called an anaplastic ependymoma, and they can spread to the spinal column in the spinal fluid.

Meningioma

Not actually a glioma, but worth including here. They grow from the wrapper of cells which cover the whole brain and spinal cord. Among the low grade versions, Grade I tumours make up by far the majority of meningiomas and most can be completely cured by surgery. That's because they're located on the outer periphery of the brain. Grade II meningiomas are more likely to come back after surgery and treatment.

What you haven't got

Many low grade gliomas will turn malignant one day (called transformation), either into a Grade III or Grade IV, or one then the other in succession. But strictly speaking, low grade gliomas are not a malignant cancer.

What we don't have is the most common, and most life-threatening type of primary brain tumour, called a glioblastoma multiforme (GBM).

This is the big bad wolf, the one that most people think of when you tell them you have a brain tumour. Sadly, their prognosis is not good. When you hear that someone has been diagnosed with a brain tumour and then they die within months, it was most probably a glioblastoma that they had.

Grade III astrocytomas (or anaplastic astrocytomas) are a malignant version of their low grade sister. They can eventually turn into a glioblastoma, but they don't always.

The other major type of brain tumour we don't have is a secondary or 'metastatic' brain tumour. These are tumours that have been created by cancer cells migrating from other cancers, somewhere else in the body. Breast, testicular, lung and blood cancers are particularly adept at creating metastatic brain tumours. Of course, these are double trouble because doctors not only have to deal with the brain tumour, but the primary cancer too. Sometimes they may not even know where the primary cancer is.

There are countless other kinds of brain tumours, both low and high grade, with countless other behaviours and treatment protocols. The area is far too wide to deal with as a single group.

I deal with low grade gliomas here because they have specific life-changing impacts, though they are not immediately life-threatening. Many of the other brain tumours, benign as well as higher grade, will have the same or similar outcomes and side effects. I hope this book offers information and reassurance to those patients too.

That's enough technical detail for now. Lets move on to living with a low grade glioma.

Write about what you know. That's the old saying about how to be a good writer. And for the last 10 years that's exactly what I've been doing: writing articles, essays, a few books and other stuff. Mainly I would write about charities, communications and ethical business. For the last two years, I've been writing about brain tumours. That's what I know these days. Living with one, dealing with possible transformation, treatment, side effects, drugs.

Write about what you know. The result is what you hold in your hands. Another thing I know about is cycling. Since university I have been in love with the bicycle. Now, approaching my late 30s, my obsession has only solidified. Long distances, road racing, challenges, time trialling. Cycling is where I belong. And it is on the bike where my own low grade glioma story begins.

I was returning home from a long cycle ride in November 2011 and was not more than a mile from home. It was a warm day and I squirted some water from my bottle into my mouth. The stream hit a broken molar tooth and all of a sudden I felt a dropping away of consciousness. It was like an electrical buzzing on the right hand side of my head, running from my face down my neck, arm and right leg.

I jumped off my bike, thinking I was about to fall over. I'd been riding hard all day and was pretty exhausted. Maybe I'd overcooked it today, and this was my body telling me to go a bit easier? The episode passed in about three minutes. I shook myself down, jumped back on my bike and ambled back home. By the time I reached my house, I'd more or less forgotten about the strange episode. It was so insignificant I didn't even mention it to my wife.

A month later, again while pushing it hard with my cycling club, it happened again. Over about 30 seconds, I began to feel a strange emptiness on the right hand side. Once again, I leapt off the bike. Cyclists crowded around me and I discovered, as I tried to tell them I was OK, that I couldn't talk. Sure, words were coming out of my mouth. But they weren't the ones I was trying to say. They were garbled, upside down, noises that didn't make sense.

When the episode had cleared, again after about three minutes, I reassured my cycling buddies. I had a broken tooth, probably with an exposed nerve. It was causing some kind of neurological reaction and I was planning to get the tooth fixed. It seemed to make sense to me at the time. After all, what else could it be?

Another month later, the same thing happened. Twice in the same ride. When I got home, I told my wife there was something strange going on. We agreed I'd go and get that tooth fixed once and for all. But before I did, I went on a cycle training camp on the island of Majorca. The cycling was great but stepping out of a sauna after a ride one day, I had another attack.

They became known between my wife and I as my 'episodes'. Because I'd convinced myself it was all about my broken tooth, I never considered going to the doctor. My dentist looked sceptical when I told him what my broken tooth was causing, but he agreed it was definitely in a bad state. Maybe even infected. After having the tooth removed, all was quiet for a while. Problem solved.

Until a month later. It was my daughter's fourth birthday when I finally admitted something was seriously wrong. I was on my turbo trainer (a kind of souped up exercise bike) when another episode came on. Somehow this felt deeper: it lasted about four minutes and brought with it some involuntary movement in my right arm and ticcing in my neck. It left me feeling weak and light-headed. So it wasn't the tooth, then.

The next day, around six months after my first episode, I finally booked an appointment with my GP. I described the symptoms, he did some rudimentary tests, asked a few questions and shone a torch in my eyes. Then he sat back in his chair with a puzzled look on his face.

"I'm not going to lie to you," he said. "I'm really unhappy about this."

Within two weeks I had been referred to a stroke clinic. Perhaps, my doctor said, I was having transient ischaemic attacks, a kind of mini-stroke that can affect younger people. The stroke doctor wasn't convinced. It took five minutes, after testing my reactions using a rubber hammer, for the rudest doctor I have ever met to tell me I was silly for thinking I was having strokes. He did, however, refer me for a series of tests: blood, an electrocardiogram (ECG) to test my heart rate, an ultrasound to monitor the movement of blood through the vessels in my neck and a magnetic resonance imaging (MRI) scan on my brain.

The MRI was the kicker. The radiographers were friendly, full of small talk and merrily going about their business. They told me the scan would take about 20 minutes. After only seven they rolled me out. They wanted to put me on another machine and give me an injection to see the flow of blood through my brain.

But their whole demeanour had changed. No more smiles, no more small talk. When I tried to glance at the screen where pictures of my brain had appeared, the radiographer physically turned me away and led me to another part of the hospital. That walk across the car park was the longest one of my life. Why, if they wanted to give me an injection, hadn't they put me on the right MRI machine in the first place?

They gave me the needle, rolled me back into another machine and the MRI began again. Afterwards I was told to wait until a doctor had taken a look at the scan. Then I was sent home.

In our kitchen, I told my wife what had gone on. We both laughed at my paranoia. After all, they wouldn't have let me out of the hospital, let alone drive home, if there was anything seriously wrong. I was due back at the stroke clinic in a couple of weeks to follow up on the tests. We let the whole thing drop for the weekend. The episodes, the MRI, the tests. The lot.

I live in a small village. The kind of place where you know just about everyone, from the postman to the pub landlord. So it didn't strike me as that strange to see my doctor, on the Monday following my Friday MRI scan, knocking at my door while I was at home looking after my kids.

He said he was just calling to see how I was and how the tests went. I realise now he was making small talk, but at the time I thought: 'How nice!' As my kids ran around, collecting leaves from the garden to give to our doctor, my GP sat on our sofa and stared at his shoes.

"It's a bit difficult with the children around, but I need to tell you that some results have come in," he said. "The MRI scan has found something in your brain. I've taken the liberty of booking you an appointment with a specialist on Thursday. And I've already written you a prescription for some steroids."

I nodded.

"I'm sorry, but I'm going to have to ask you not to drive until you see him."

My doctor never actually said the words. But the truth hung in the air between us so ominously that it didn't even need to be uttered. I had a brain tumour.

Everyone has a story to tell about when they first discovered they had a brain tumour. For some, it began with a big bang: a debilitating seizure or blackout. For others, the symptoms crept up on them over a number of years. This book contains testimonies of over 20 low grade brain tumour patients who have been kind enough to share their stories for this book. Here we meet just a few of them:

"The haemorrhage happened at about 11pm one night when I was in bed. I suddenly and out of nowhere felt the worst pain I had ever experienced to the left side of my head, like I'd been struck with something really hard. I ran to the bathroom as the pain was making me nauseous and shouted to my flatmates. They were in bed but ran to my side and the three of us sat on the bathroom floor while I was in agony. My flatmate Laura called NHS Direct, and crushed up painkillers for me to try and swallow. She was concerned when I said the water she gave me tasted really strange: she told me later a relative of hers had said the same thing when having a stroke."
Angela, 24, pilocytic astrocytoma Grade I

"I found out on Christmas Eve at my mum's. I went round to prepare for Christmas dinner, went upstairs to vacuum and decided to pluck my eyebrows (like one does). I woke up on Boxing Day evening, having had three days of seizures in A&E. I had a scan and they found the tumour. They then found a scan from three years ago, also showing the tumour! That hadn't been diagnosed, despite my having neurological issues, some loss of the use of my leg and being told I was bipolar because my moods were swinging."
Amber, 48, oligodendroglioma Grade II/III

"When Tyler was 12 he started being very sick at night with the most awful headaches. We were initially told that these were migraines. But I got him seen at the local hospital because I knew it couldn't be a normal migraine. There was no preparation for being told there was a mass on his brain. I think I went into shock but Tyler just went very quiet. The surgeon explained that Tyler was seriously ill. His dad asked what our options were. The surgeon replied with the words that are engraved on my heart: 'If he doesn't have this surgery he will die'".
Janice, mother of Tyler, 16, glioneuronal tumour Grade I

"About 13 years ago I happened to be working in a hospital teaching IT to medical staff, when I suffered two major fits, one straight after the other. When regaining consciousness I was somewhat disoriented. It took a little while to understand where I was, in a bed in hospital. I was given a scan and was told that I had a brain tumour, probably a low grade glioma."
Richard, 55, anaplastic astrocytoma Grade III

"I had a two-year-old and a newborn and had been getting headaches and had a lump on the top of my head which was tender. I was turned away from two different doctors; they said I was just tired with the baby and I must have banged my head. I knew something wasn't right so got a third opinion and by chance this doctor's husband had been recently treated for a brain tumour, so she was clued up. Scans showed I had a 7cm meningioma which had compressed my brain and eaten into my skull because it was so big – hence the lump!"
Lindsey, 35, meningioma Grade I

"I had no idea I had a brain tumour. I was 58 and had not been ill, but had high pressure in my eyes that was causing some problems with my eyesight. It was my eye specialist who sent me for a brain scan. He then telephoned me at my workplace and bluntly told me I had a tumour. I was very shocked, especially as my mother had died from a brain tumour 38 years earlier. I was working in a fairly public place and was surprised that he told me in such a manner. My colleagues were very supportive and sent me home, where I had to tell my family. It was a very strange and difficult Christmas that year."
Jenny, 65, meningioma

"I had no previous symptoms. I got up to drive to work as normal and was on the village roads about 6.30am. Two minutes after leaving my house, I felt a huge surge of something between pain and a 'freezing' of my left side which I just could not fight against. I though it was a heart attack. I was fighting to control the car and the next thing I remember was being on the wrong side of the road. The first reaction was that I was still alive which was good! Once at home I sat on the settee and I had another seizure, so my wife called an ambulance. I remember being in a removed state, as if I were looking in at events. At hospital I had another seizure and I was placed in an induced coma. The next I knew I woke up in a ward that turned out to be intensive care."
Rory, 41, oligodendroglioma Grade II

In it for the long haul

On the Macmillan Cancer Support charity's website, there's a special talk board for people affected by low grade brain tumours. At first I didn't understand why the topic was called 'In it for the long haul'.

Two years on from diagnosis, it makes a lot more sense. When I walked out of the consultant's surgery on the day I was officially told my diagnosis, I didn't think I'd be alive today. I went home to prepare my will, to be with loved ones and in some senses to wait to die.

It was only slowly, and with much of my own research, that I came to properly understand that far from an immediate death sentence, having a low grade brain tumour can often be more about living than dying.

The ironic luck we have is that our brain tumours are unlikely to end our lives quickly: instead, living low grade is about the daily drip-drip-drip of the tumour's emotional and physical effects on us and our families. Living for today, dealing with and adapting to our tumours, is what living with a low grade glioma is all about. We truly are in it for the long haul, and when our long haul finishes – well, then our lives will change considerably and there will be new issues to deal with.

So how do we get on with the life we do have?

For some of us, our lives will be relatively unchanged. Perhaps only marred by the knowledge that there is a time bomb in our heads that one day might go off. For others, we will have monthly, weekly, even daily side effects that need to be controlled, managed and accommodated into our lives. By us and by those around us.

For some, their tumour might have been found by accident – as a result of an MRI scan for a completely different reason – and they might not have yet had any negative experiences at all. Treatment for them, if any, might be aimed at knocking the tumour back so it's even longer before any problems show themselves.

For many of us, our low grade gliomas are likely to have been sitting there for many years. Once upon a time my tumour was just a microscopic cell gone haywire. Given that low grade gliomas can grow at a rate of a couple of millimetres or less a year, there's every chance my tumour has been around since I was a teenager, perhaps even a toddler. It had grown to bigger than a kiwi fruit before it started making its presence known.

Whenever I'm feeling particularly miserable about my life expectancy, I think about that microscopic cell to help me through. Imagine, I think, if treatment can set the tumour back to toddler size again? Suddenly I feel like I have my whole life before me.

Lumping it all together

One of the most frustrating things about having a low grade glioma has been a feeling that some of my doctors have seen so many low grade gliomas, they tend to send us packing just to get on with our lives. As if our lives haven't been changed forever.

The side effects of having a tumour – both emotional and physical – have often been sidelined. Those episodes I was having on the bike turned out to be partial focal epileptic seizures, a direct outcome of my brain tumour. My neurologist (brain doctor) has prescribed increasing doses of anti-epileptic drugs. But apart from that, the impression I've been given by the medical establishment is that the rest just isn't their problem. As one consultant oncologist put it to me when I complained about the headaches and speech problems I was having: 'Well, you're bound to have side effects aren't you.

You've got a brain tumour.' She then left the room, the consultation over.

For low graders, the symptoms and side effects of our tumours are often the key problem we have to live with. Yet as far as I can see, they're the very thing that some clinicians find least important. That's some other people's experience too, but certainly not everyone's.

> "I found out that me and my tumour were second rate, there was nothing seriously wrong with us and we were wasting these important people's time. This has happened time and time again with different doctors or specialists who are all very interested until they find out it isn't cancer or life-threatening."
> *Paul, 58, meningioma low grade*

> "I have found the doctors to be understanding of the process and have made things as easy as possible at each consultation. By being open to questions it has allowed me to understand why waiting has been the right option, and conversely when moving to another step and why."
> *Duncan, 33, astrocytoma Grade II*

If you've been prescribed anti-convulsant drugs, steroids or other medicines to help keep the symptoms of your low grade glioma at bay, you'll be familiar with reading the little thin leaflet that comes in the box along with the pills. Take a look at the side effects of the drugs, and you'll often find those listed seem to be exactly the ones you were experiencing before you even took your first tablet.

This medicine may cause drowsiness, fatigue, seizures, changes of mood, irritability, depression, memory loss, temporary loss of vision, poor balance, dizziness, and more and more and more... One prescription I take has such a long list of possible side effects, I get the impression that stubbing my toe might just be down to the drugs. And worse still, the very act of reading those lists of side effects made me suddenly notice things about my health I hadn't quite noticed before. So, I've taken to ignoring the side effects list on drugs.

After all, if you have to take the drugs to keep your tumour in check; and your doctor is reluctant to deal directly with your side effects; and you're not sure if you're imagining the side effects anyway; well who cares whether it's the tumour itself, the drugs, or simply the stress and anguish of your condition that is generally buggering up your life? It's all part and parcel of being a low grader.

I've decided that my tumour, its side effects and the side effects of the drugs, might as well be lumped in together. They're all part of a low grade glioma. They're all part of my condition.

Changing diagnosis, changing prognosis

At the time of writing I'm likely to live longer than I thought I would a couple of years ago. But in a few months time, that might change. Then I'll be expecting to live less long that I expect to live right now.

Confused yet?

A feature of low grade gliomas is that while there may be long periods of relative stability, our diagnosis (a description of our condition) and histology (the type of tumour we have), and therefore our prognosis (expected life span) can change over the life of the tumour.

That's a strange position to be in. For many cancers a diagnosis brings with it a slightly clearer prognosis, a well trodden treatment regime and some relative certainty. (I say relative, because nothing in cancer is certain.) For low grade gliomas things certainly don't work out clear cut. That can be a blessing, but can also bring stressful confusion.

If you're avoiding information about life expectancy and brain tumours, you may wish to skip this section.

Anyone who has looked into the life chances of those with low grade brain tumours is likely to come away with less certainty than they had before they started. And that's not just because the figures on survival in low and high grade gliomas are so variable and are influenced by so many factors. (See Prognosis)

The key issue for those of us living low grade is that as consultants find out more and more about our particular tumour, their diagnosis can become more precise. The more precise their diagnosis, the more the estimation of our life expectancy can leap from one extreme to another.

When I was first told I had a brain tumour, that was as much as I knew. And while it wasn't an official diagnosis, it was enough information for me to go away to research the likely outcome. But I researched on the internet, where there were wildly differing opinions and figures. I was in a panic and wanted as much information as I could garner. (What follows is what I originally found. You should turn to the chapter on Prognosis for more accurate and less panic-driven information).

On my reading, my long term-life chances were pretty slim. For malignant brain tumours in adults, my Google search told me, only just over a third are still alive a year after diagnosis. And only 15% live for more than five years. I didn't even know at that point there were low grade, benign, high grade or any other subtype of brain tumour. I just found the worst case scenario and it was enough to strike paralysing fear into anyone.

A few days after my GP first told me of my tumour, I went to see a brain tumour consultant. After examining my MRI scan, he told me he strongly suspected ('I'm 99% sure') that I had a low grade (Grade II) glioma.

With that information my prognosis suddenly and dramatically improved. According to my research, the median survival rate for glioma patients was between five and eight years. That meant 50% of patients were still alive five years later. I was facing a significantly improved life expectancy from when I walked into his office that morning. It comes to something when you *celebrate* the fact you could have only five to eight years to live, but that's what it felt like coming away from the hospital that day.

Then things changed again a year later. After an increase in seizures, and an apparent uptake of blood in my tumour, my neurologist said – with what felt like the same level of certainty as the other consultant had used the year before – that my tumour was very likely transforming into a high grade glioma (a Grade III).

Once again, my life expectancy had changed. According to my clumsy late night internet surfing, half of Grade III glioma patients are still alive one year later and just a quarter after two years. So I was back in the danger zone again.

The neurologist advised me to have a biopsy, to confirm his suspicions and to get an accurate idea of my tumour type. Following the biopsy, the surgeons did not find any Grade III cells (though they couldn't confirm there weren't any in the tumour somewhere). So I was officially classified as a Grade II again, and back to the better figures once more – a median survival rate of 11 years on my reading.

But the news was better still. The type of tumour I had was called an oligodendroglioma. That carries with it a life expectancy better than some of the other types of low grade glioma tumours. Now, my median life expectancy had improved again.

Two weeks later, I learned that the particular genetic

makeup of my tumour meant I was far more likely to respond to radiotherapy and to particular types of chemotherapy than if I had different genetic markers. That made my prognosis yet further improved, to a median life expectancy of 14 years, according to my layperson's research.

There was, later, a suspicion that my Grade II tumour was building more of its own blood vessels, something which would put me back in the Grade III camp. My life expectancy would change again, and I'd have to start treatment soon. As it turned out, at the time of writing, the tumour is stable, so I'm still a low grader.

In a sense I'm lucky. Since that first visit by my GP, my life expectancy appears to have – apart from a few blips – generally improved. Others may find theirs has taken the opposite trajectory. Many of us, I suspect, would have found their diagnosis change, then change again, then change again. But there will be some low grade glioma patients who get a certain diagnosis from day one that never changes.

But even all this isn't the end of the constantly changing imbroglio of living low grade. That's because there are so many other contributory and confusing factors in brain tumours. Any life expectancy estimations we do make don't actually provide that much information. They present more questions than answers.

When we talk about life expectancy, do the figures mean from when the particular diagnosis of a low grade glioma was made? Or when a suspected diagnosis of a more general glioma was made? The difference might be technical, but the result could mean an extra couple of years at least. And that's a lot when you think you're going to die.

And what about the statistics on life expectancy of gliomas? Does that include those who are later given a more precise diagnosis? Or have they been taken out of the equation because they're not simply *general* gliomas any more but something more specific? And what about surgery? I can't have surgery, so that reduces my chances. But then again, I'm very fit, relatively young and my tumour is not so big that it is yet making life difficult to lead. These are all positive prognosis factors.

What you end up with, if you try to play this good-score bad-score game, ends up looking like one of those massive equations brain box mathematicians have on their blackboards. You try to add up the positive factors, subtract from them the negative factors, and you come up with an approximation that is so inaccurate you might as well have not bothered.

And why not? Because life expectancy just doesn't work that way. Turn to Prognosis to understand why.

How to deal with constant change

The nature of low grade gliomas is that – in effect – in exchange for a better prognosis we live in a limbo of not quite knowing what's going to happen next. Or when that next something may happen.

Our expected survival rates can never be particularly accurate. They can constantly change as our condition develops, and they're often no more certain than sticking your finger in the air to guess which way the wind is blowing.

The question then becomes: how do I deal with this uncertainty? Though it's easy to come away from each doctor's appointment with a temporary euphoria or despair, I've found those extremes very quickly settle back into a generalised feeling of just not knowing. It's difficult to take, but all of these wildly differing factors are why our doctors are reticent to give us accurate estimations of what will happen to us. They're not hiding something, they simply don't know.

I've tried to stop second-guessing my tumour. Doing so

won't change the ultimate outcome, it'll just make living with it yet more stressful. I've learned to take the temporary highs and lows for what they are, but to appreciate the generalised hum behind them as one of constant uncertainty.

Of course, the apple cart is frequently upset because friends and family, as well as strangers, tend to want to know your prognosis. It's hard to explain how complex it all is. Many don't understand how it can change so wildly up and down, or how the condition can fluctuate. They can be surprised when they see you one month and you're having lots of problems, then when they see you again you're in tip-top condition.

This is where very good friends can support you the most. They offer you the time and a receptive ear to explain the detail. They work with you to understand why it's so hard to respond to the question: 'How long have you got?' We low graders are in it for the long haul, and to properly understand how it all works our best friends need to be in it for the long haul with us. For the rest? Well, I just say that doctors don't know. I'm taking every day as it comes. Cliché it may be, but I sometimes have to tell myself that too.

Managing uncertainty, managing hope

The fact is that none of us know what is to come. We know it could be bad one day, but we don't know how, we don't know when. How do you carry on with that knowledge?

Uncertainty has become the background noise in my life, always there like a quietly ticking clock. Every now and then it annoys, then you forget about it for a while. The kids need to be taken to school, the lawn needs mowing, there are visitors to clean the house for this weekend. I've learned to live with uncertainty about my future with the strategy of trying to put it out of my mind and by tackling it when it rears its head.

But every now and again, you're reminded. The dentist wants to book an appointment in a year's time, and you find yourself asking: 'Will I be having treatment then? Will I even be alive?'

A friend calls you up and asks if you want to go on a cycling holiday with them next year. Do you say yes right away? Or do you procrastinate, just because you don't know how good your health is going to be?

I spent the first year after diagnosis almost paralysed by this uncertainty. Sure, I got on with the day-to-day things, but I found it very difficult to think long-term. I refused to plan holidays, to book appointments or dates in the distant future. Even an invitation to a party or dinner in two months seemed like a lifetime away. There might be more important things to think about before then.

Until one decisive day I told myself I would no longer live that way. The year gone by had already proved I could be in extremely good health. How many opportunities had I already missed because I had refused to commit?

Instead, I decided I would not assume I would be unwell, but the opposite. I would assume I would be well, and not go into treatment, nor die in the near future. I would go ahead and plan. I'd say yes. I'd commit. The tumour was already controlling my present, I wasn't going to allow it to control my future too. If things did take a turn for the worse, then I would deal with them as they came. And if they did, would anyone begrudge me that cancelled dinner date or missed dental appointment?

Every now and again that uncertainty creeps back in. My wife and I find ourselves asking: 'But what if?' Then we remind ourselves that we can't live our lives according to what might happen, only by what really is happening right now.

"When it comes to longer-term plans the challenge and decisions are so difficult. The nature of the illness means some can live a long life, while others can pass suddenly. It is impossible to know which category I fall into, hence the uncertainty for the future. If we delay plans, there is no chance of leading a normal life. On the other hand, if we go ahead with big plans, like buying a house or having children, what would be the effect if my health deteriorated?"
Duncan, 33, astrocytoma Grade II

There's an old phrase that seems to encapsulate lots about living with a low grade glioma: you've got to go there to come back again. Many of us have to go through the process of knowing our health will deteriorate, maybe even end before we'd expected. We need to grieve and face that abyss, before we can come back and get on with our lives. It's easy for others to tell us not to worry about the future. That we should put it out of our minds. After all, you're not dying yet.

But my experience has been that it was only after taking the space to fully contemplate what had happened that I was able to come to terms with my diagnosis and put my life back together. I had to go through a short journey of peering over the precipice, before pulling myself back and rebuilding my life as far away from the edge as I could.

Battling your brain tumour

But what about fighting? What about bravely battling my tumour? What about being determined to win and not to die? To not allow my glioma to beat me?

For some people, this fighting talk is part of dealing with their diagnosis. Some honestly believe they can beat their tumours. Perhaps, some achieve it. Others use the language of battling, knowing it is a conscious strategy for dealing with what they really know is inevitable.

Both approaches are entirely understandable and I commend anyone who feels that approach works for them. The approach I've found most helpful might be regarded by some as resigned. Even nonchalant. For a long time, I've been quite philosophical about my condition: what will be, will be.

I know that one way or another, my particular type of low grade glioma is likely to end my life. I know there will be physical and emotional pain, for me and for those I love. Am I scared? Yes, of course. Am I angry? Yes, I'm livid. But right now I'm not dying, I'm living. There are enough side effects and emotional pressures to deal with. I'd rather worry about them, than what may or may not happen in the future.

Others will have a different approach. Those of us living low grade are as diverse as the tumours in our heads.

> "Mostly my tumour feels like one of those old rusty bombs that's sitting at the bottom of the Thames doing nothing, never likely to explode. I've only been living with it for two to three years though and it is a big deal. But in reality, life is very easy to get on with as usual."
> *Ben, 37, oligodendroglioma Grade II*

A kick up the backside

I'll never say I'm pleased I got a brain tumour. I hate it and I wish every day that it hadn't happened. But it did happen. My family and I, just like your family and you, have to deal with it. We will all be dealing with it long into the future.

I'm not grateful for having a brain tumour, but I do recognise that it has reminded me about what is important in my life. It has encouraged me to spend more time with my children and my wife, to look at each day afresh, to exercise more and to eat more healthily.

Most of all it has encouraged me to really follow my fundamental passion: writing and telling stories. Since diagnosis, I've written a regular blog about living with a low grade brain tumour and cycling. I've written this little book. I've written books, articles and creative pieces on a range of other subjects that interest me.

They just about make me a living, but they also make me happy. When life is suddenly in shorter or more uncertain supply, wouldn't you rather spend more of it happy and following your passions, if you can?

When you've recently been diagnosed with a brain tumour, you don't know which way to turn. You may not know what will happen in the future. Or even how to deal with the present. I am no life coach. I can only speak from my own experience. And mine has been one of retreating to the things that make me happy, that I am passionate about, that I feel really make up the essence of *me*.

This strategy helps to put the bad things out of my mind. Or at least into some perspective. In some cases, things I initially thought were important about my tumour have faded into the background because I'm too busy getting on with my life. For me living low grade is about understanding and concentrating on the good things I do have in my life, and then making the most of them.

2

Symptoms and signs

IF YOU READ the leaflets on brain tumours, clinicians and charities generally separate the side effects of having a low grade tumour into two types: symptoms and signs.

Symptoms are things you feel yourself, which might not be apparent to the outside world. Things like mild seizures, headaches, tiredness, weakness on one side of the body or confused thoughts.

Signs are things others might notice, but which may or may not be apparent to you. Major seizures, changes in mood, slurred or confused speech, bumping into things, forgetting the names of everyday objects.

For some, these symptoms and signs might be the reason you went for a doctor's check-up in the first place. Seizures and headaches are the biggest driver of that initial visit to the doctor. Sometimes their failure to clear up after we've first been sent packing by doctors is the reason we keep returning to tell them there really *is* something wrong.

The nature of brain tumours means every patient will experience different symptoms and signs, or none at all. It all depends on exactly where your brain tumour is located, how big it is, and how invasive it is into the healthier brain tissue surrounding it.

"Nanette suffers from tonic-clonic seizures. Normally she gets a warning sign in her left hand which enables her to press her Lifeline button before she loses consciousness. She then thrashes about and they can last from five to 10 minutes. Other times she has absence seizures which give her no warning. She does have falls and we wonder whether these are caused by absence seizures. Due to her disability she is unable to get up off the floor by herself, her left leg stops working which also causes her to fall."
Jen, mother of Nanette, 38, oligodendroglioma Grade II

"My life is hardly affected by this tumour, I have not had one seizure since it was discovered, my oncologist and neurologist say I am not likely to ever have a seizure because of it being at the front of my brain and not being too large. I gave in my driving licence and now have it back two years later. I take 1,000mg of anti-epileptic pills every day. They have no discernible side effects whatsoever."
Ben, 37, oligodendroglioma Grade II

Seizures

These have been the most pronounced sign and symptom of my brain tumour, and are the most frequent side effect of low grade gliomas seen by doctors. When tumours grow they press on parts of your brain that don't usually come under so much pressure. So our brains don't quite work like they should.

Seizures due to brain tumours are essentially epilepsy. For me, they don't involve any serious convulsing: the fall over, shaking unconsciousness kind of seizures we often assume epilepsy is all about. That makes it difficult when I tell people I have epilepsy, because this tonic-clonic fitting is what people expect you to mean. For some low graders, tonic-clonic seizures are exactly what they will have. But for others, seizures will be very different.

Mine are more like mini-fits known as partial focal seizures: they include mild convulsing, weakness and a kind of emptiness or absence in a single, or particular parts of the body. In my case, they're down the right hand side, particularly in my arm and hand, and also in the right of my face. I've discovered that in most people it is the left hand side of the brain that controls the right hand side of the body. No surprise then that my right-focused seizures are caused by the tumour in the left hand side of my brain.

On the day I'm writing this, I expect to have around 10 to 15 seizures. I did yesterday, and the day before. The deep seizures I was having when I was first diagnosed, those that used to come on when I was pushing hard on my bike, are very different to the light seizures I most often have these days. That's thanks to my medication. They may be more frequent, but the drugs I take have dampened down their intensity. That doesn't mean they're not annoying, but sometimes I barely notice I'm having them. Occasionally, the seizures do get deeper for long periods: I report that to my neurologist and he often increases a dose of one of my drugs and things calm down again.

My seizures are so unlike anything I've ever experienced, it's hard to put the sensations into words. For my own use, I've started to use a convenient short-hand for defining their intensity.

My *light* seizures feel like an electric buzzing in the right hand side of my mouth, particularly in the teeth. Remember the whole broken tooth affair? I also get a metallic taste in my mouth and even a feeling like there's a light ball of chewy electricity at the back of my tongue that I can't quite bite down on. There's also a slight feeling of absence or lightness in the right side of my brain. Often, it's accompanied by pins and needles in my right arm and hand. The whole episode builds up over about 30 seconds, then ebbs away again just as fast. I've found these seizures so light I can continue a conversation, typing or riding my bike without having to stop or anyone really noticing anything is up.

Medium seizures are just like the light ones, only they feel slightly more intense. The pins and needles stretch down the right hand side of my body, particularly in my right arm and leg. The emptiness in the right of my brain feels, well, emptier. And the buzzing and metallic taste in my mouth is more pronounced. It feels like the right hand side of my face is pulling down, as if the muscles there have given up. But a mirror check has shown this is just a sensation, rather than real.

The key difference is that medium seizures affect my speech. I know what I want to say, but the words come out just a little garbled. Sometimes I'll stop mid-sentence even though in my head I'm continuing to speak. I'll trip over my words, as if my brain is churning them out quicker than I can put them together. Sometimes there are odd words and sounds shoved in where they don't belong. These seizures last about a minute or two.

Deep seizures are something else entirely. It was these that first took me by surprise when I was cycling hard, and eventually sent me scurrying to the doctor asking if I was having a stroke. Over about 30 seconds, I'll gradually feel consciousness on the right hand side of my brain simply drop away, and the whole of the right hand side of my body go weak and unable to move. If I was cycling, there was no way I could stay upright. Sometimes, I've sat on the floor just to be safe.

The tingling and pulsating in my head, again on the right side, feels intense and the chewy metallic feeling on my tongue very pronounced. I swallow a lot, and my speech is either garbled or I can't speak at all. Strangely, songs pop into my head from when I was a kid: nursery rhymes, pop songs, poems. But when the seizure clears, I can never remember what they were.

There's also a strange feeling during a seizure of having experienced a few of these sensations before. A kind of: 'So, that's what that was!' It's as if when I was younger I'd occasionally had similar sensations, but never paid much attention to them. Whether this is simply *déjà vu* playing tricks or something connected to the earliest growth of my tumour I guess I'll never know.

But, even with the deepest seizures, I've never fallen unconscious. I'm very aware of everything going on around me, watching from the left hand side of my body as the right goes into free fall. These deeper seizures take about a minute to really set in, they last between three and four minutes, then slowly ebb away again. Sometimes they come in a couple of waves. The last thing I regain, sometimes up to seven or eight minutes later, is my speech.

Light, medium or deep. It's no surprise doctors have taken my driving licence away. Seizures have become a daily part of my life, and almost an internal measurement of how my tumour is progressing. My neurologist says there's no reason to believe worsening or more frequent seizures are always indicators of tumour progression. But they *can* be indicative of exactly that. And that's why I keep a close eye, to see if we can tally them up with any changes on my MRI scans.

"I coped very well for about 12 years on medication to prevent having fits. In late 2009, while running, I suffered minor fits without really realising what they were and I didn't take much notice. In May 2010, I suffered a severe fit while out running and after consultation with my neurologist and surgeon, they decided to operate."

Richard, 55, anaplastic astrocytoma Grade III

Speech difficulties

The other key indicator that something is wrong up there is that I frequently have speech difficulties (dysphasia) even when not having seizures. This is another often reported indicator of brain tumours because they can press up against the parts of your brain responsible for processing language and producing words. It doesn't happen all the time, but it does feel like my speech problems have gradually worsened since diagnosis.

Often, it's just not quite being able to find the right words: 'Can you please pass me the, er, you know, the [points, waves his hand in the general direction], the, er, magazine?' I always get there eventually. At least unless someone I'm speaking to finishes my sentences for me, which happens a lot. (I haven't quite decided if that annoys me, or helps me out.)

Sometimes, too, I repeat words in sentences. They're usually the words running up to the main point of what I'm trying to say: 'Oh, we really ought to, ought to, ought to clean the windows.'

One thing I don't notice much, and nor has my wife, is something my friends have told me I do. I run my words together, without a gap between them. It's as if I'm slurring from being drunk. I think my wife and I don't notice because we live together and hear each other talk every day. But friends who don't see me often say they notice a difference.

"The impact of strokes on my speech was that I suffered from expressive dysphasia, where words are mixed up or forgotten even if I've said them two minutes before."
Paul, 58, meningioma low grade

"I'm not a big fan of speaking to a crowd as it exaggerates the stutter I've developed. I know that won't help me to overcome it. In school, I used to do plays in front of large crowds and loved it. Perhaps one day I'll try to make myself better at that."
Angela, 24, pilocytic astrocytoma Grade I

Headaches

I've been lucky enough to experience only light headaches. For other low grade glioma patients, headaches have been so bad they've not been able to get out of bed, tolerate light or go outside. Unexplained extreme headaches are what lead many low graders to seek out medical investigation.

On a bad day, I might feel a tight band around my head or a pulsating pressure, this time on the left hand side at the temple just where I know the tumour is located. But I know these sensations may just as much be down to my imagination as to the tumour itself. And certainly my doctors have never reacted with any concern about them as indicative of anything except my own paranoia.

It's no surprise that increasing pressure in the brain from the tumour itself, or from swelling around it, causes headaches. There's only so much space up there, and with the skull keeping it all in there's no escape when it gets cramped. For some, the headaches are unbearable.

"At first her headaches were caused by a build up of fluid surrounding the brain which caused pressure in the front and back of her head. Steroids were supposed to help, but when trying to come off them the headaches became worse. One time she ended up in A&E with fever and a severe headache. The only relief was painkillers and sleep. Now we've been told the cause of the headaches is probably the scar tissue from all the operations she has had. The pain management team recommended paracetamol and codeine phosphate together which seemed to work. But sometimes the headaches still last for days."

Jen, mother of Nanette, 38, oligodendroglioma Grade II

Tiredness

This isn't a big side effect for me, because as a keen cyclist I can never really tell whether my fatigue is down to my tumour, the drugs or simply my spending a lot of time doing exercise.

Nevertheless, some mornings – maybe once a month, and particularly after changing my drugs dose – I do wake up feeling so tired that I have to go back to bed just after breakfast and will maybe wake up an hour or two later. I'm usually groggy for the rest of the day. And maybe every two weeks or so, I'll hit a tiredness wall around 4pm. I'll again retreat to bed, usually for an hour in which I feel my body is resetting, and I wake up fresh to continue the evening.

"I need to sleep a lot, and often get an overwhelming urge to just lie down and sleep. Sometimes the urge feels almost uncontrollable. I can't count the last Saturday or Sunday when I didn't at least have a half-hour nap."

Angela, 24, pilocytic astrocytoma Grade I

Personality change

Because the brain is responsible for our personalities and the way we behave, a tumour pressing on a particular part of the brain – usually the frontal lobe – can cause us to act in a different way than we did. And it can change how we behave as it grows.

Once again, the drugs prescribed for seizures can cause very similar personality changes. So it's sometimes difficult to know what is the medication and what is the tumour. Side effects from radiotherapy and chemotherapy, which may cause your tumour or the area around it to swell, can also create these personality changes. Those with low grade brain tumours report becoming more irritable or aggressive, becoming apathetic, having mood swings, losing their inhibitions and behaving in unsociable ways, like swearing in public.

It's often partners or friends who notice the change before the patient does. A visit to the GP can help get you counselling or therapy, or sedatives and other drugs to help things balance out a little.

> "My personality is an area that my wife and daughter see a lot more than me and they describe my short temperedness and anger as serious problems. They have both said I am not the person I was."
> *Paul, 58, meningioma low grade*

> "As regards personality changes, I'm easier to lose my temper but it's better now than straight after the operation. I get frustrated easily; upset, sometimes to the point of tears, but again not as much as straight after the operation."
> *Richard, 55, anaplastic astrocytoma Grade III*

This is all something my wife would definitely recognise. On bad days, I seem to find even the most trivial things annoying. It's like my tolerance level for life has reduced by a good few notches. I can get more irritable, even a little moody. With my children I occasionally have a shorter fuse than I'd like to.

Interestingly, when I'm moody or argumentative my wife sometimes claims that's down to the tumour or drugs. That of course does nothing to diffuse my irritability because in my mind what I'm annoyed about *really is* annoying. It feels like she's downgrading whatever irritation I have. (When I pointed this out to her she reminded me I used to say exactly the same things to her when she was pregnant. Fair point.)

It's worth noting here that my irritability and moodiness was most pronounced, even debilitating at times, when I started taking anti-convulsant medication. After all, before that MRI scan and before popping that first pill, my personality was all sweetness and light. Honest.

Such personality changes and brain function changes are one of the worst things for partners and loved ones to cope with, while you yourself may not notice the difference. In the long term, a permanently changed personality can be devastating for you and your loved ones. The closeness, intimacy and shared experiences that brought you together in the first place may sadly be lost. In short, you just may not be the person you used to be. But simply knowing the changes are down to the tumour, rather than a *real* change in your own or your partners' personality may somehow make it easier.

What else?

For me, there are a few other symptoms and signs I experience which could be down to the tumour itself, or the drugs I take. Or maybe they've always just been part of me, but my diagnosis has made me notice them more.

I have, for example, a generalised feeling of weakness down my right arm and hand. Some days it's worse than others, but it feels as if that arm isn't as strong or useful as my left. Another thing I've noticed is a clumsiness I'm sure I never had before. Things seem to slip out of my hands a little more readily than they used to, and I occasionally bump into doorways with my shoulders. Do I also trip up and stub my toe more often too?

So, where now with side effects?

For many low graders, it'll be the symptoms and side effects of the tumour that are most annoying in the short term, though of course the longer-term implications can't be dismissed. While my doctors have not tended to worry about my symptoms, or just throw more drugs at me, I've sometimes felt dismissed by that approach. For me, living low grade is all about these small but noticeable changes in our lives. We do have a right to feel as well as possible, even if our lives are not immediately in danger. The brain tumour charities seem to understand this very well, but the medical establishment – in my experience at least – seems slower to catch on.

Headaches, seizures and nausea can be temporarily dealt with by more drugs. Other avenues, like speech therapy or physical manipulation, might help with speech problems, balance, weakness or clumsiness issues. And there are any number of complementary and alternative medicine (CAM) approaches which many cancer patients – though I'm not one of them – say help them to deal with the day-to-day symptoms of their illness.

But sooner or later, when seizures become unmanageable using drugs alone or those headaches can't be controlled by the pills, there really is only one way to go. That tumour is going to have to be made to shrink somehow. And that means treatment. Since many low grade gliomas can never be cured, many patients will have treatment to remove as much of the tumour as possible, to slow down or inhibit its growth, but also to reduce side effects. Treatment can increase (sometimes for many years) the amount of time tumours take to grow back to a size where side effects show themselves or come back.

Adapting to side effects

One way or another, side effects will often be something we have to put up with. Often, it has to be a case of adapting our lives so the side effects we have are easier to bear. That sometimes takes significant life changes, as well as emotional hurdles to clear.

> "I have to go to quite a few hospital appointments, so I have to incorporate those into my working life and schedule them into my diary. I always carry sunglasses with me everywhere now, even in winter, as my eyes are so sensitive to light: I'm scared of suddenly finding myself somewhere really bright and not being able to open my eyes properly. I also get tired. I do feel sad that I need to rest sometimes, like when my nieces are over and just want to play. I've missed out on hours of quality time with them when they're over to visit."
> *Angela, 24, pilocytic astrocytoma Grade I*

> "I have found adjusting to the hearing loss hard. If I am in a noisy environment I can't hear what people are saying. I have no idea what direction noise is coming from and it does affect my balance. I try to lip read, but it's a little hard still."
> *Nicola, 35, acoustic neuroma Grade I*

The side effects I have had started off as worrying health issues that would send me running to the doctor. They then became just a pain in the backside. Now I have got so used to them that, unless they're particularly bad, they barely affect my life at all. That's not because they're not there any more. It's because I've got used to them and I've adapted my life to accommodate them.

Take seizures, for example. When I started having them in front of friends and family, I would leave the room embarrassed. But all I left behind was a concerned and uncomfortable silence in the room while I was gone. Once I got more used to them, I decided to take a different approach. If I had become dependent on a wheelchair, or had lost my sight, I wouldn't try to hide that from my friends and family. I wouldn't scurry away from them because of my disability.

So I started to stay put when seizures came on. My family and friends got used to them too. Now the conversation or activity carries on, albeit with me playing a temporarily reduced part. When the seizure has abated, we all continue as if nothing has happened. Very quickly my seizures were accepted as just part of all of our lives, not something that should be dealt with by me alone.

These days, if I know I'm going to be spending a lot of time with people who don't know about my seizures or my brain tumour, I try to explain as early as I can. I'll ask people to just carry on if, temporarily, I'm unable to speak properly. To spare their sanity, I don't tend to reveal my brain tumour to every single person I meet. It can come as quite a shock. Often I'll just say I have a mild form of epilepsy and not to worry if I go a bit strange for a while. Epilepsy is a term most are familiar with, so we can all just get on with our lives.

Emotional impacts

The emotional side of experiencing side effects is also something we have to adapt to. The biggest thing for me, particularly at the beginning, was that seizures and speech difficulties were a constant reminder that I had a brain tumour. I might be able to go for a few hours at a time without thinking about the cells slowly growing in my brain and their eventual implications. Then suddenly I'd have a seizure and it came like a body blow: Oh, that's still here.

That might ruin my day, or at least make me feel depressed for a time. So far, I've never reached a dose or mix of drugs that have removed my seizures altogether. But they don't bother me in quite the same way as they did and they're not a constant reminder of my brain tumour. They've just become part of my life.

> "As for the paralysis I'm struggling with this, I feel like a freak even though I know deep down that I'm not. I feel people stare at me. I'm extremely self conscious and won't have my photo taken any more. It took a while to adjust to changing the way I have to do things because of the paralysis and I hate looking in the mirror as it reminds me of everything. I will be relieved when I can look at myself without feeling and seeing so much pain."
> *Nicola, 35, acoustic neuroma Grade I*

Before we got the drug dose just about right to make my seizures lighter, I would have deep ones frequently when riding my bicycle. For someone who had spent much of his life on the bike, and even raced it from time to time, this has had an enormous emotional impact. In those early days, I had to give up racing completely and couldn't even ride in a big group. I just wasn't a safe bet for my fellow cyclists. I'd sometimes be reticent to even go out on my bike because I knew I was likely to have a seizure at the side of the road.

To have something that was such a big part of my life taken away, almost overnight, made me extremely unhappy. It can't have helped my irritability much either. In the end, I decided that I wouldn't allow the seizures to dictate my cycling life. Instead, I would try to adapt. Trying to stay on my bike became a motivation.

To start with I began spending more time on my turbo trainer in the garage. No danger of falling off in front of a car there. I also went to my neurologist and other doctors, and demanded that they took my seizures more seriously. My doctor may have been satisfied that the drugs were reducing my seizures, but that wasn't enough. I wanted to be able to cycle with a group again, and that became the marker *for me* about whether the drugs were working.

I also talked to my cycling friends about my seizures: asking if I could still come out with them, what to do if I had a seizure and the risk they were taking (not much). My seizures, I explained, were quicker to clear than it takes most cyclists to fix a puncture. By finding ways to accommodate and adapt to my seizures, with friends and the people I cycled with, I was able to stay on the bike. Instead of allowing it to bring me down emotionally, I channelled that challenge into determination. I had no choice. Either find a way to get back on the bike, or suffer the frustration, even depression, I knew I'd experience without it.

I can now continue riding even in a big and fast moving group of cyclists. In fact, I've even been able to take up road racing and time trialling again. In this, I know I have been lucky. Others will have side effects they are unable to control and which might entail more drastic life changes than mere adaptation and determination. That could be anything from introducing disability adaptations, moving house, having to be accompanied wherever you go, leaving a job or starting a different one, or claiming some kind of benefit. All of which may sometimes bring their own stress, feelings of negativity, disappointment and even poor self-worth. Your GP, charities and the Citizens Advice Bureau may all be able to help with information and guidance, adaptations and making any emotional impacts easier to deal with.

I deal with some other emotional impacts of brain tumours elsewhere, and many of the ideas and experiences I share there apply just as much to the side effects of tumours as to dealing with the diagnosis itself. But it is worth repeating: for low grade glioma patients, the side effects we experience, as well as the emotional impact that those side effects have, can be the most significant part of our disease. Sometimes – at least in the short term – they're the only part of having a low grade brain tumour that matters. Finding ways to adapt and deal with their impact should be at the top of our agendas, and certainly should be higher up the priority list for our doctors.

3

Life challenges

SO A LOW grade brain tumour and sometimes its eventual implications present one big source of stress and emotional turmoil, and often physical problems too. But there are also other implications which present real life challenges. They too are part and parcel of living low grade. They may not be the tumour itself, and they may not be physical side effects, but they are important nevertheless. And so they too are part of our diagnosis.

There are obviously lots of life challenges involved in having a disability or any kind of long-term illness. I've not tried to outline them all here, but rather ones that are particularly pertinent to those with low grade gliomas.

Driving

Most people diagnosed with a low grade brain tumour will suddenly find they have their driving licence taken away, at least to start with. If you have had an epileptic seizure of any kind, it's almost certain you will be banned from driving. The rules are pretty complex, and worth checking in full with the charity Epilepsy Action.[1]

In the UK, the Driver and Vehicle Licensing Agency (DVLA) prevents anyone who has had an epileptic episode during the day or night from driving for at least 12 months after their last seizure. To get your licence back, you have to show you're not still having seizures, you're following your doctor's advice on drugs and precautions, and the DVLA has to rule that your driving would not be a danger to the public.

If you only have night seizures, or if you have partial or focal seizures that leave you able to act and don't make you unconscious, you have to show that pattern consistently for a year before you may be allowed to drive again. If you've ever had an unconscious seizure, the period is three years. The DVLA needs a detailed description of what happens to you before they'll give your licence back. And of course, there are acres of forms to complete.

It's a difficult day indeed when you have to package up your driving licence and send it away with a sad little form to the authorities saying you're no longer allowed to drive. It may be hard to take, but it really makes sense. Either full-on tonic-clonic seizures, or partial focal seizures could create a real danger if you're behind the wheel, hammering along the M6 at 70mph.

But for many of us, driving is a pretty big part of our lives. Whether getting to work, taking the kids to school or the swimming pool, going on holidays or simply enjoying a drive, being banned from doing so can present significant problems. For low grade glioma patients – some of whom may never be able to drive again – being banned from getting behind the wheel isn't just a damned inconvenience. It can effect our very sense of self.

There's something about being able to drive, even having a *right* to drive, that is an intricate part of our lives. Take that away, and it feels like a little part of who we are has been taken away too. And in a very real way, particularly if you live in a rural area or depend on your car for work, being banned from driving is truly disabling, even if you don't actually have a physical disability.

But what to do about it?

It seems pretty clear to me that I'll never drive again, so frequent are my epileptic episodes. But I think I'm one of the lucky ones. I already worked from home most of the time, I'm used to travelling around by bike, I love rail travel and my kids' school is within walking distance. And there's a bus that leaves every half an hour not far from my home, though it does only go into town or into the near wilderness in the opposite direction.

What I have found particularly difficult is that I can't just pop to the shops or out to the zoo with my children without the faff of getting on one or more buses. It can be so demoralising to envisage a mammoth journey on public transport. It feels unfair on both me and the children. Sometimes it has been downright depressing to feel trapped in our own home.

But there are a couple of things that I have done to make life without a car slightly easier. It is perhaps something I've found easier to adapt to than other aspects of living low grade (though adapting to my wife's driving has been something of a challenge). I've more naturally taken to the bike when I've needed to go places; I've got used to forward planning what journeys I need to take; I've turned more to the internet to do shopping; and my wife has been generous with her time driving me and the kids around.

"I hated the loss of my driving licence because it meant the loss of my independence, though my family were very supportive. When my licence was reinstated, I paid for one proper driving lesson to boost my confidence. This was three years after my operation, by which time the correct medication for my epilepsy was established and I had been seizure-free for two years. I know I will be on this medication for the rest of my life and will have to renew my licence every three years."
Jenny, 65, meningioma

"I am so dependent on my parents. Most 26-year-olds are living on their own with a job; I am currently at home looking for a job, asking for lifts if I want to go anywhere."
Rachel, 26, neurocytoma Grade III

Getting back on the move

There are a number of provisions made for people who are unable to drive because of medical conditions. I've found a mix of my free bus pass, discounted rail travel, as well as savings on car insurance has saved our family hundreds of pounds since I was first diagnosed. That makes not being able to drive a little easier to bear.

The provisions made for those banned from driving because of epilepsy are not unsubstantial. But they can't and won't suit everyone who is used to driving or needs to for work. At the time of writing, if you are prevented from driving because of epileptic seizures, you can apply for a pass that gets you on to any bus in the UK completely free. I am also entitled to a Disabled Persons Railcard. While this does cost a small fee, it paid for itself in a couple of journeys, particularly because my wife gets a third off too when she travels with me. In some circumstances, my train pass also allows me to travel as an off-peak passenger during peak times.

Also at the time of writing, if you are on a low income or on certain benefits and are willing to jump through some hoops, you can qualify for reimbursement of any car and taxi travel expenses to get to hospital and doctor's appointments.

Work

If you are employed, a significant impact of your changing health situation is bound to be your job. There is, of course, the practical side of having to build your condition into your employment, adapt to any changes in your ability to carry out your job and to accommodate any time off you need for MRIs, doctor's appointments, treatments or even surgery. Add to that the attitudes and needs of your employer, and the problem of work becomes yet more significant.

But living low grade is not just a case of adapting your work to your condition, or your employer adapting your job. My diagnosis led to a complete crisis about what I was doing with my life. Did I even want to continue my old job? Was I even capable of it? Was it still fulfilling, knowing what I now knew?

I am self-employed. Before my diagnosis, I worked as a trainer and consultant to the charity sector on writing, media and marketing. I also ran a series of events and workshops for charities. I employed other writers and project managers frequently, and had a satisfying, relatively profitable business as well as an excellent work-life balance.

But when I became aware of my condition, one of the first questions I asked myself was: Is this really what I want to do with my life? If I do only have a short time left, what other things would I like to do that I haven't done? Suddenly, I found I no longer quite fitted into the work-shaped hole I'd carved out for myself.

As a self-employed person with a little money in the bank, I was lucky enough to be able to give myself a six-month sabbatical from work. It allowed me to really consider what to do next. Go back to the same work? Write that book I'd had turning over in my mind? Work in environmental conservation? Something completely different? I also had that terrible six-monthly-chunks issue to deal with. What if I decided what career I did want, then in six months time was told I'd have to go into treatment? Or that my life might be in danger? Where would I be then?

After my six months off, I decided to pack in most of my old work and to write a book. It was an itch and while I didn't earn much of a living from it, I was glad to have scratched it. But after that – around a year after diagnosis – I hit a barrier of complete despair. It was probably my lowest point since diagnosis. Just what was I going to *do* with my uncertain future?

The extreme lack of direction made me incredibly depressed. I'd start then stop a project. I'd make a decision to do one thing, then give up after a couple of weeks. I had no confidence to apply for jobs, but wasn't particularly bothered about going back to my old work either. At the time of writing, I'm still not sure where I'm going. I wonder whether low graders ever really do. I've started to pick up some training and consultancy again, and am satisfying my writing itch by working on projects like this book.

Again, I'm incredibly lucky to have been in this position of choice. Many patients simply don't have a choice. They either have to continue working in their old jobs, or to stop working altogether because of their condition. For other low graders, the continuation of their work has provided the only enjoyable, consistent and diverting part of their diagnosis.

Work is a significant part of all of our lives, so it's no surprise that living low grade can involve considerable change and reflection in this area.

> "I've not worked since diagnosis. I loved my job and I was filled with drive and ambition for my family and had a competitive edge. These drivers are now gone. I still do not know what my reaction would be to work even if I were able to return, as my motivations are no longer there."
>
> *Rory, 41, oligodendroglioma Grade II*

> "When going for a job I feel I should tell them about my condition because with my job you are looking after someone's child, the most precious thing to that family. If you start off being open and honest then hopefully that is good. Yet due to most people's lack of knowledge on the subject of brain tumours the worst is immediately assumed. You can almost hear them thinking: 'Oh my god is she going to drop down any minute?' It isn't ignorance, but just the unknown."
>
> *Rachel, 26, neurocytoma Grade III*

> "I only recently told my manager that there was anything wrong. I was two months into the job before I told her. It was a case of finding the right time and place, but also a case of wanting to prove myself, being able to show what I'm capable of without being handled with kid gloves. When I told my manager, she actually said she thought I was amazing and gave me a big hug."
>
> *Angela, 24, pilocytic astrocytoma Grade I*

If you are employed, it might be tempting to throw in

your job and tell the boss where they can stick it. But I found a sabbatical a better option. Any boss with the slightest sympathy ought to give you at least some time to digest what's happened. They may even consider paid compassionate leave.

As sympathetic as any employer is going to be to our change in circumstances, they still have a business, a charity or a public service to run. And that means there will be difficult decisions to make. But employers can't simply just turf employees out because they have epilepsy, cancer or a brain tumour. Some patients have challenged and won employment tribunals based on exactly these issues. This book can't be a guide to your employment rights, nor the benefits those with long-term illnesses may be entitled to. Some of the larger cancer charities and the Citizens Advice Bureau have reams of information for those looking for help and practical support in these areas.

Looking back, I don't regret taking the time off from work. But I do regret chucking in my old career, letting old contacts go and discontinuing the events I used to run. In hindsight, I realised, I quite enjoyed the work. I also think it could have provided some stability, even if it wasn't what I definitely wanted to do in the future. I wish I'd not been so hasty and kept my options more open.

This isn't a self-help book. I'm not going to tell you anything is possible. But I certainly found my diagnosis forced a little clarity in my life. It encouraged me to consider whether I was doing what I truly wanted to do. Though I've still not found the answer I'm glad I've taken the time to explore what I'd really like to do now that things have changed forever.

Medication

Here's something you may not have been told by your doctors. It takes time to get the medication right. For some reason, we expect drugs given to us by medical professionals to work exactly the way we imagined they would: bring down swelling, ease those headaches, reduce the seizures. It's as if taking a pill is going to allow us to carry on our lives as before. And that just isn't the case. It does take time for doctors to find the drugs that are going to work best for us. There are dozens of epilepsy and anti-convulsant drugs. Every person's brain tumour is different, a different size and in a different place. What drugs work for one patient may not work for another.

Our doctors don't know until they've prescribed something, though they ought to have some kind of idea. The drugs then need time to bed in before a picture can be gathered of whether they're working or not. Doctors will want to give medication for weeks, or even months, to see whether they're working or whether they should try something else. We all want quick solutions, so this waiting can certainly be frustrating.

After being diagnosed with a low grade tumour, I was almost immediately prescribed an anti-convulsant drug (levetiracetam). I was started on a low dose, which was gradually increased until I'd reached a higher dose on to which I was supposed to stay. The drugs did nothing, absolutely nothing, to stop the seizures or affect their frequency or intensity. But the doctor waited for a good six months before agreeing to look again at my medication.

When my seizures started coming much more frequently and much more intensively, my neurologist added another drug (clobazam) which was supposed to calm the seizures. They did, for a while, but then they came back. So he increased the dose. It calmed down again, but then came back stronger than ever. Eventually, he added yet another drug to my daily dosage (lamotrigine). And gradually increased the dose of that.

There are three important things to note about my

experience. First is that even this drug cocktail – 10 pills every day – has not completely controlled my seizures. I still have waves of weeks when I'm seizure-free, followed by weeks with seizures. The drugs appear to have changed the pattern, and reduced the problem. But they've not eradicated it.

Secondly, don't take away the idea that my current dose of particular drugs will work for anyone else. Our body makeups are different. We don't do the same amount of exercise. We don't eat the same foods. We have different tumours. We have different brains.

Thirdly, brain tumour patients should not be afraid to approach their consultants to talk about their experiences with drugs, to ask questions and ensure their voices are heard. There can be a tendency for us to elevate doctors to know-all beings and to assume we should just do what we're told and not ask questions even if we don't understand. My experience has been that if you do seek explanations, doctors are often very willing to explain their thinking. Asking questions actually felt empowering, like I had some control over my future.

One thing my wife and I found useful was to keep a daily spreadsheet of my drugs and tumour side effects. Every day we recorded the doses of the different drugs I was on, and the number of daytime and nighttime seizures I had. What we ended up with was a graph showing my different drug doses as they were increased, and the frequency and intensity of seizures as time progressed. From it, we could see the seizures increase, then decrease, in response to my medication.

We discovered that my anti-convulsants could actually make seizures worse before they got better. No-one ever told us that. We'd had to figure it out for ourselves. But it helped us to prepare every time my dosage was increased.

The seizure diary was something concrete I could email to my neurologist ahead of meetings or at other times when I was worried. At a glance he could see the pattern of my side effects and the drugs I was on, and that assisted him and saved time when we met. In a sense we could *talk the same language* about my experiences. He could point to peaks and troughs on the graph and try to explain them. He could tell me what was normal and what was not. I found it gave me a greater understanding of the drugs I was taking, and the effects they were having (or failing to have). My neurologist was pretty impressed too.

> "I hate taking drugs, they silently control your life.
> Some in the morning, some in the night with the odd blood test thrown in to check your drug levels in your blood stream."
> *Marie, 35, astrocytoma Grade II*

The other key aspect of medication when living low grade is that there may be an awful lot of it. That too doesn't come without problems.

First, I found, was the difficulty of remembering what to take and when to take it. Considering some low grade gliomas create memory loss, what chance do we have? The answer, of course, was a weekly pill box. They come with chambers with days of the week marked on them and for each day, they split into four separate containers: morning, noon, evening, bedtime. I got mine from a 99p store.

But that pill box still has to be filled once a week, which brings with it another pain of living low grade. I can only get a few weeks worth of medication at any one time. I have to remember to re-order and then return to the pharmacy every other week for one of my drugs, because they only prescribe it in doses of 14 days at a time. I also have to try to keep track of what other drug refills I need. It takes considerable brain work and forward planning, again something that is occasionally lacking in brain tumour patients.

If I go on holiday, things can get even more complex. I have to work out what drugs I'll need while I'm away, ensure I have sufficient quantities to get me through the holiday and remember that I'll need some for when I return. I have to order them in time to get them for the holiday and then, after all that, remember to actually pack them in my luggage.

I always take a copy of my prescription and my doctor's telephone number when I go away too. Coming off drugs suddenly can cause problems, so I wouldn't want to be stuck abroad without them. And anyway, a copy of my prescription would surely reassure any customs officer who opens my bag and sees the sheer quantity of drugs I'm attempting to take out of the country.

Getting support

> "I rely a lot on Facebook brain tumour groups for support and I've made some good friends, got help and comfort. My cancer unit runs a monthly support group for brain tumours which is also great."
> *Amber, 48, oligodendroglioma Grade II/III*

We all need support in the weeks, months and years after diagnosis. The levels of support and their type will change, but we shouldn't feel we have to go through living low grade alone. I found asking for support the most difficult part. That first call to a brain tumour charity. That shy attendance at a support group. But once I'd done it, a world of assistance opened up to me. The following are just some of the support avenues available.

Clinical Nurse Specialists

From the medical side of things, low grader's emotional support is supposed to come from your Clinical Nurse

Specialist (CNS). They're expert nurses in cancer or even in brain tumours, and will be a first point of contact between you and your consultant. I've found them very good because they have seen a lot of what you're going through before and will share with you any experiences they've had. Unfortunately, not all NHS trusts provide low grade tumour patients with a dedicated CNS.

Family and friends

Your partner, if you have one, is likely to be the closest source of support for you. But they will also have their own support needs. Try as I might, I know I'm not the best person to offer support to my wife.

But over the weeks and months, I've been able to gauge the reaction of other family and friends, and who I'd most like to turn to when things get tough. That's sometimes someone to moan or even cry with. Other times, its a hand with babysitting or advice on my finances. As well as getting the support they provide, I know I'm giving them a chance to *do something* too.

Charities

There are a number of very large cancer charities, a handful of larger brain tumour charities, and lots of very small brain tumour charities. All of these can offer some kind of support emotionally, as well as practically, and have lots of information about the different kinds of brain tumours.

My personal experience has been that Macmillan Cancer Support have been very good regarding helping me to understand my financial and benefits situation (applying for free bus passes, disability benefits). Cancer Research UK have been extremely good with the information they provide about technical aspects and diagnosis. The Brain Tumour Charity has been extremely supportive in terms of both information, access to materials to help with fundraising and in making me feel part of the 'brain tumour community'. The charity brainstrust have been very good with their emotional and information support, particularly the 'brain box' of information they send to those who are newly diagnosed. Some friends have raised money for the third largest charity in the field, Brain Tumour Research.

I've found a lot of the smaller brain tumour charities less helpful in a supportive role. They're essentially fundraising charities set up in the name of a lost loved one. However, they are an important and vibrant part of the brain tumour community. They offer confidence that there are many others out there with the same experiences as you, who care and want to do something about brain tumours.

There are a wealth of organisations out there, all providing their own particular services. In a sense, this is a shame because it can be confusing who you should go to if you need information or support. I've sometimes wished there was one port-of-call that would deal with all of my needs. But at other times, I've welcomed the diversity of services offered.

Support groups

Most often supported by charities, there are a number of face-to-face brain tumour support groups which meet across the country. Some are organised around NHS services and can provide medical information, others are wholly separate and provide only emotional or mutual support.

The support groups offered by brainstrust, for example, are informal meet-ups over a pizza. They're an opportunity for those affected by all kinds of brain tumours, and their families, to meet up, socialise and share experiences in a very informal setting. In contrast, support groups offered by The Brain Tumour Charity tend to be slightly more formal, with groups meeting at hospitals or community centres. The Brain

Tumour Charity also offers formal information days across the country, at hotels or conference centres, with speakers and panel sessions about new research and initiatives, as well as opportunities to share family and patient experiences. Alongside being a great source of concrete information, the coffee and lunch breaks offer an informal way to meet other brain tumour patients and experts.

> "The Kent group has been a great help to us all. A Macmillan co-ordinator, two patients and two carers make up the steering group. Whenever our speakers have heard the stories from members, they are usually overwhelmed. But they're also surprised at how happy everyone is to be at the meetings. We have had some sad times but on the whole there is a great buzz."
> *Jen, mother of Nanette, 38, oligodendroglioma Grade II*

In the same way, there are a number of online forums that offer discussion and support. Macmillan Cancer Support runs one specific to low grade brain tumours (called 'In It For The Long Haul') at its website, while The Brain Tumour Charity has an online forum for patients, family and friends. This diversity of ways to get group support is important. An online community perhaps offers an opportunity to be bolder and ask questions you may be embarrassed about asking in person.

But not all support groups are the same, and not all are as helpful as you might hope. In one group my wife went to, the guest speaker there stated that those who thought positively about their condition, and who turned up to support groups like this one, were more likely to live longer. This simply isn't supported by any scientific evidence and was challenged by a few of the attendees. My wife came away feeling worse than when she went in, as well as angry and frustrated.

Helplines

There are currently two dedicated brain tumour helplines, run by two different charities. There are also helplines specific to whatever side effects you may be having: epilepsy, weight gain, loneliness, depression. At the end of the phone line is likely to be someone who is trained to listen, to offer information and in some cases advice or counselling. A helpline can be good for quick specific questions about your condition, side effects or rights and benefits. But they're also good for those just feeling a little lost and who need someone to talk to.

My experience has not been consistently good. I've received useful information I didn't know on the one hand, which has left me more knowledgeable and confident about my condition. But I've also been told to look on the internet or go and see my doctor. For one number I called, I felt like the person on the other end of the phone was going through the motions and wasn't helpful at all. But perhaps they were just having a bad day.

> "I found the telephone support line at one charity not very helpful as mine was a low grade tumour. But a small telephone support group helped a lot, spending long periods talking to me. Cancer charities did not want to deal with me as my tumour was not cancer which made me feel left alone to get on with coping and a fraud for seeking help."
> *Paul, 58, meningioma low grade*

Counselling

As the whole of this little book makes clear, being diagnosed with a low grade glioma is likely to bring with it immense fear, turmoil, uncertainty, depression and confusion. For those particularly struggling, a range of counselling may be available on a formal and informal, paid and free basis.

My own GP offered my wife and I counselling during one of the earliest follow up meetings I had with him. Because it came with a GP's referral, I got six 50-minute sessions as well as a first taster session on the NHS. The meetings were with a trained counsellor who would not refer back anything I said to my doctor, and was only obliged to pass on information if they thought I might put myself or others in danger. My counsellor was happy for me to access my six sessions as and when I needed them, and we ended up meeting every three weeks or so. Hospices often offer counselling too, even to those without immediately life-threatening or life-ending conditions.

There is a social stigma attached to receiving counselling or therapy, so to begin with I didn't tell many people I was doing it. But I found it immensely helpful. It offered the opportunity to talk to someone about my condition and feelings who wasn't emotionally engaged with my situation. Of course our family and friends *say* we can speak to them about even our darkest thoughts, but in reality we're very likely to tell them what they want to hear or what we think they can take. With a counsellor the deal is different: they're being paid to listen non-judgementally. To gently probe, to help draw out main points, but otherwise they are understanding, sympathetic professionals there to hear what we have to say.

I talked with my counsellor about a whole range of things, from my feelings of frustration about my diagnosis and some of my doctors, to the way I feared for my wife and children's future. I talked about annoyance I had with some friends and family about their reaction, and practical things like the difficulty of juggling work and childcare with hospital appointments. I wasn't offered any 10-point-plans or told to meditate or burn incense sticks. I was just listened to, got a few things off my chest and was made to feel relatively normal.

Practical ideas

One of the biggest worries for me in the months following my diagnosis was what would happen to my kids if I suddenly had a serious seizure while I was out in town, alone with them. So with kind neighbours, I organised a phone tree.

I wear a wristband telling people about my epilepsy and providing two emergency telephone numbers. They are for people who can either come to assist themselves or, if they can't, have the numbers of other people who have agreed to assist. All in all, there are eight people on my phone tree. At least one should be able to get to me and ensure my children are safe. I've never had to use my phone tree, but I'm very glad it's there.

Complementary and alternative medicine

I include complementary and alternative medicine (CAM) as support, rather than in the section about treatments, because there has never been conclusive evidence that CAM can cure brain tumours or reduce their symptoms. They're not medical interventions, and it is illegal in the UK to promote anything to cure cancer that doesn't actually do so.

However, some people do report that CAM helps them to deal emotionally with having a brain tumour and that it *relieves* their symptoms. Proponents say undergoing CAM treatment has helped them to relax, feel physically regenerated, deal with any pain and to come to terms with their diagnosis. The most popular strategies for relaxation and easing symptoms are meditation, massage, reflexology (applying pressure to the feet, hands or ears) and acupuncture (penetration of the skin with needles to stimulate certain points on the body).

In the spirit of openness, I must disclose that I am a CAM sceptic. I concur that they can act as a placebo, essentially making you feel better because of the action of doing it rather than any ingredient. From my perspective, if there are no negative health effects then there's probably no reason why patients shouldn't consider CAM. But to think it offers anything like a cure is misguided.

There are a number of specialist books and websites about complementary medicine, cancer and brain tumours. The charities Penny Brohn Cancer Care, CANCERActive and Yes to Life are considered specialists in this area.

Travel insurance

Travel insurance presents the usual dilemma for low grade glioma patients. We just don't know what's going to happen in the near or distant future, and that affects whether or not we can get reasonably-priced travel cover.

When I was first diagnosed it was from an MRI scan alone. I hadn't had surgery. I knew that I'd have to disclose my diagnosis to insurers, even though I hadn't had a confirmed diagnosis from a doctor. But even with that rather woolly information, I quickly discovered that many mainstream insurers wouldn't touch me. Or else they ramped up travel insurance costs so much the insurance cost as much as the holiday.

After seeking advice, I went to one of the specialist travel insurance companies that deal with cancer and other chronic illnesses. Cancer charities tend to have a list of these. From a specialist cancer insurer, after filling in acres of forms, I was able to obtain travel insurance at a reasonable cost. Though it certainly wasn't as cheap as it had been before diagnosis.

It was after my biopsy that things got really tricky. That's because I had to tick the box that said I'd recently had brain surgery. Let's be realistic. What insurer is going to back someone who's had brain surgery in the last year? The online quote systems – even those from cancer cover specialists – all refused to give me a price. Instead, they suggested I call their office to discuss in more detail. For which I read: talk to us and we'll say no. Or we'll find ways to ramp up your quote so high we might as well say no.

And there was another box to tick on those forms too. Are you likely to have treatment for cancer in the next year? Well, that's just the problem with low grade gliomas isn't it? We just don't know. We may well have an MRI pretty soon that suggests we do need some kind of treatment. If a travel insurer has paid up after something going wrong on holiday, and then you subsequently go into treatment, wouldn't they be asking for their money back? Or pursuing you for dishonest form filling?

In short, low grade glioma patients are unsafe bets for travel insurers because we don't even know ourselves what the future may bring. And that means higher premiums or refusals to cover us at all. In the end, I gave up trying to get travel insurance for the first year after my biopsy. And I've concluded, because I live from six-month scan to six-month scan, I'll never be able to say I won't have treatment in the next year. The most I'll be able to do is ask my consultants to write a letter stating treatment was *unlikely*. I'm hoping a letter like that might do the job of getting me reasonably-priced premiums. But I'm not crossing my fingers too tightly.

And while we're at it: life insurance. If you've been diagnosed with a life-threatening brain tumour, particularly a low grade incurable glioma, it's just not going to happen. Unfortunately for those who didn't have life insurance before they were diagnosed, we're a little stuck with that fact. Financial advice charities may be able to help with ways to work around insurance requirements for borrowing money or getting a mortgage.

"Insurance is the area where I have had a particularly difficult challenge. When buying a house, in order to get the mortgage we wanted, life insurance was required for both myself and my wife. For my wife this was no problem, while I was unable to get any cover due to having a pre-existing medical condition. Although this is something we have been able to get over, it has led me to question how many people have life insurance before they end up needing it. Prior to needing the cover, I had never considered life insurance as a priority. I think many 30-year-olds would be in the same boat."
Duncan, 33, astrocytoma Grade II

4

Family and friends

APART FROM MY wife, I hadn't even told close family about the strange seizures I was having until I'd started medical tests to see what they were.

On the day after my first MRI, but before my doctor had told me I had a brain tumour, I told my brother and his wife I'd been having the episodes and that I was having some tests to find out what it was all about. We talked about the possibility I was having mild strokes or had a blocked artery leading to my brain. It never occurred to us it might be anything more serious.

When my doctor turned up with the news of what my MRI had discovered, the first person I called was my wife. She was miles away working, but she decided to head home straight away. I then called my brother.

"My doctor has just turned up," I said. "I've got a fucking brain tumour."

"You're joking," he replied, which where we come from

doesn't mean 'you're joking', it means: 'Oh shit, that's really bad news'.

It wasn't a difficult conversation. My brother and I have a very good relationship and I wasn't nervous or fearful of telling him. It was just information I had to impart. I was a little tearful, so was he, but otherwise the conversation was quite practical. I shared the basics, and he asked me if I was ready to tell my parents.

I decided I wouldn't speak to them until my wife had got home. We spent hours talking and trying to understand what had happened. The information from my local doctor was very sketchy: he wasn't a specialist, but he was reassuring. At that stage none of us knew anything more than it was *likely* to be a brain tumour.

My doctor booked me in to see a specialist close to my wife's parents' home a few days later. We decided to tell her folks. We'd need them to take care of the children while we went to the hospital. We didn't talk about it much with them because apart from a very hazy idea that something serious might be wrong, there was nothing else to say.

I decided not to tell my own parents until after that specialist meeting. I wanted more time to absorb the information myself. I didn't want them to worry unnecessarily, but nor did I want them to start spreading the news – as I knew they would want to – to other members of the family. It was only after the specialist hospital meeting a few days later, where I learned I had a suspected inoperable and incurable low grade glioma, that I called my folks. I first phoned my brother to update him, but by that time we'd both expected the news I'd received.

"Bro, you're going to have to tell Mum and Dad," he said. He offered to do it for me, but I knew it was something I had to do for myself.

I phoned my mum from outside the hospital. I simply gave

her the headlines of what the specialist had told me: I had an incurable brain tumour, the better end of the bad ones, how the whole thing had come about, that I'd been banned from driving and we'd take another look with another MRI in three months. There was nothing else to say. She agreed to tell my sister, who lives close to her. We shared a few words of reassurance and left it there.

I then phoned my dad and had the same conversation. When we arrived back at the in-laws, we had the same conversation again. My wife and I had decided to get the bus home, rather than be picked up, and we just held hands and stared out of the window trying to take it all in. For a few more days, we decided to keep the news quite close to our chests. We wanted time to digest what was happening, before news started spreading, as bad news inevitably does. It felt like news that belonged to me, and I was strangely possessive of it. So possessive, in fact, that I was quite annoyed when my sister posted about it on her Facebook.

After a few more days, I decided to call my closest friends. I drew up a short list, many of whom I hadn't spoken to for a month or so, each of us busy just getting on with our lives. In the end, I made three calls and saw one couple in person. I then realised I couldn't do it that way any more.

Each conversation would start with the usual chit chat, as if I'd called up just to say hello. I'd then have to find an opportunity to slip in, as we were sharing the latest updates in our family, the words: 'Well, I'm afraid there's something I have to tell you. I've been diagnosed with a brain tumour. It's the better end of the bad ones, but, well, you know, it's not good news.'

Having that conversation was so painful and so stressful each time. I would pick up the phone and my heart would beat faster, my mouth would go dry. I knew I was sharing heartbreaking news that I hadn't come to terms with myself.

Eventually I took the coward's option. I wrote a one-page briefing on what had happened and how it had come about, life expectancy and the information as I then understood it. I then composed a short email, copied to all of my friends and extended family, and pressed send. The tone of the message was carefully crafted to indicate we weren't necessarily up for long telephone calls, but an email or card would be welcome. The email I wrote was as follows:

"Good morning. Sorry to be the bearer of bad news on a wet Tuesday morning and sorry to do this by email. If I haven't been able to talk to you personally so far, please accept my apologies. Things are kind of busy just now.

"On Thursday just gone, I was diagnosed with a brain tumour. It was discovered after an MRI scan I had as part of a series of tests I had lined up because of some strange 'seizures' I was having while out cycling. While the tumour is essentially incurable and will end my life, I'm not at death's door just yet.

"With some luck, I should be around bothering you all for a good few years to come. I'm working (if you can call what I do working) for the next three weeks, then taking six months off. I'm feeling pretty philosophical about it just now, Sarah is in bits (she, [my daughter], [my son] and you guys will be the ones left behind after all).

"I'm keeping this short and sweet, but I've written a short briefing about what I have, which I've attached and should go some way to filling the information gap. It would be good to hear you are thinking of us, and

74

to see everyone in the really near future. Sorry to break it like this, and love to everyone."

Many friends said it was very typical of me to write a briefing to share the news. By laying it all out clearly, they said, it had helped them to quickly understand what had happened, its seriousness, and provided the answers to many of the questions they had.

You mean you're not dying?

A difficult hump to get over when telling friends and family about low grade brain tumours is the immediate assumption that you are about to die. Or at least go into serious treatment pretty soon. But that often isn't the case. When I first heard I had a brain tumour I also put two and two together and ended up with five. So my friends were likely to do the same.

All of us assume a brain tumour most often means death pretty soon after. When I told someone, I often found myself immediately following up with something along the lines of: 'Don't worry, I'm not dying just yet', or 'Don't panic, I've had it a long time and I'm likely to be living with it for a good while yet'.

People just don't understand brain tumours (or any cancer really) until they are directly affected, and they certainly don't know there are different types, with different prognoses, different side effects and that their impact can often depend on where they're located in the brain. So I started to gather a few stock facts about my condition to share when the response I got from friends and others was sheer panic.

"It wasn't the medical profession that seemed to distinguish between low grade and high grade tumours, but the outside world. I could sense that people felt great relief when I told them it was low grade as opposed to something that was highly malignant. One mother actually said to me: 'Oh, that's alright then.'"

Penny, mother of Harry, 17, juvenile pilocytic astrocytoma Grade I

Among people I didn't know particularly well, the reaction I received was most often embarrassment. After all, what do you say to someone who has just told you they have an incurable condition? Particularly if you don't have long to talk or the opportunity to share much detail. Among these people, many said: 'Oh god, I'm sorry' and then went into awkward silence, simply not knowing how to continue. I found either changing the subject, or offering the broad headlines about my condition was the best way to deal with this. They'd then ask more questions, or most often check in next time they'd see me (probably after they'd done a Google search).

In other cases, people I've told have reached around for some words of reassurance, but tied themselves in knots. Sometimes they have mentioned someone they knew who had a brain tumour but just as they're speaking have realised that the story ends in that person's death. They then kind of trail off without finishing.

My usual response is to ask what kind of brain tumour they had, whether they'd had treatment and then how things had ended up. Then I've offered sympathy if the news wasn't good. It excuses them from the guilt of having to tell me the worst case, demonstrates I'm not too afraid to talk about the implications of my own tumour, and shows them that there are a range of brain tumours and that mine might be quite different.

"Normally when I tell someone I have a brain tumour it stops them in their tracks and you can see them looking awkward as they don't know how to handle this information. I then add that it is low grade, slow growing and benign so it could be a lot worse. That seems to ease the situation a little bit."
Rachel, 26, neurocytoma Grade III

Who else to tell and how?

After my biopsy, while I was carrying around a three-inch scar on my relatively bald head, I received a few jokey comments outside my children's school, from people in shops or on the bus along the lines of: 'Oh, what have you been doing with yourself?', or 'Has the wife been giving you the knock around?'

How do you respond to those you barely know who have inadvertently gotten themselves into deep water? And at the same time, do you even bother telling people about your condition if you have nothing outward at all like a biopsy or surgery scar to indicate anything is even going on?

It took some getting used to, but I generally approached the problem 007 James Bond style: the information was available on a need to know basis only. That meant the random person on the bus was told, with a laugh, that it was just a little surgery scar and I left it with that. If I was to have a serious seizure, I hoped, my emergency information wristband would provide all they needed to deal with the immediate situation.

"I am always cautious about telling people, as one time at university a lady asked me why I had been away. I told her and she fainted right there in front of me! I had to get her a chair and some water and sit

with her until she felt better. After that, I'm always cautious of telling people at the right time and in the right place."
Angela, 24, pilocytic astrocytoma Grade I

For some people I'd see more regularly I'd generally tell them the truth. Just not the juicy detail. I took the *biopsy - brain tumour - don't panic* approach. In a way, I hoped they'd pass the detail around – say at the school gates – so I didn't have to keep on having the same conversation. And indeed this is exactly what did happen at my kids' school. I had to let some of the teachers know about the diagnosis, treatment plan and how we were dealing with telling our children, which I did formally in a letter. We were worried our kids would find out by accident at school something they hadn't properly understood at home. We also asked for a little flexibility in time off for our kids, in case of hospital appointments.

> "Always, always, always keep the teachers totally in the picture. They will work with you (in our experience anyway) and need to know what is going on so that they can adjust the way they deal with your child without it looking like favouritism."
> *Penny, mother of Harry, 17, juvenile pilocytic astrocytoma Grade I*

The members of my cycling club also needed to know something, particularly that I was at risk of seizures when I was out on my bike. I started by talking only about epilepsy, only later letting more information trickle out. Eventually enough was out there that most of my cycling friends knew about the seizures, as well as what was causing them. Some would chat to me about it and ask questions. Others accepted the information, and we just moved on.

Having a low grade brain tumour is a huge part of my life. But it's not the only part, nor the sum total of me. I never wanted to be *that guy with the brain tumour*, but I realised I was more likely to become that if I allowed the news to circulate behind my back. Better to be part of the conversation, I decided, so I could offer accurate and reassuring information.

And one more strategy I found helpful in communicating with friends, family, acquaintances and even people I didn't know was this: to remember that life isn't all about me. As much as my tumour was part of my family's experience, and even a juicy little bit of news that people might want to share, it didn't mean I should always be the centre of the conversation. Others have their own lives, their own problems, their own kids and their own news.

When someone asked how I was, or what was the latest development in my condition, I made an effort to quickly follow up by asking something about them. How were they doing? How were their kids getting on at school? Were they planning a holiday any time soon? I tried to demonstrate the same level of interest in their lives as they had shown in mine. It helped to normalise the brain tumour as part of my life, and helped me see further than my own narrow experience. It was also just good manners.

Taking these approaches, I found I became *that guy with the brain tumour* for only a very short time among everyone I knew. Soon after, I just became *that guy* again.

The impact on your partner

If you have a partner, a very close best friend or a close sibling, you may find as I did that their experience of your low grade brain tumour is just as intense, painful and confused as yours. It's too easy to imagine the brain tumour affects only you. In our own grief and fear for our lives going forward, there may sometimes be a tendency to forget how our diagnosis affects those around us, particularly those who love us the most.

It's an old cliché in cancer circles, but there is some truth to the idea that it may be even harder for your partner (or close friend etc.) than it is for you. After all, we're the ones who are dealing with the practical side of things: the surgery, the treatments, the side effects and of course, if it comes to it, the actual dying. While we're too busy getting caught up in the technicalities of our condition to get too stressed or emotional about what has happened, our partners have a whole gamut of fear and emotions to go through, often without so much distraction. For them, perhaps, the impact is a lot more emotional and painful, yet much of the time they feel they have to be strong and not show their distress, because they're supposed to be supporting us. What a terrible place to be in.

Among low graders I've spoken to there has been a range of reactions from partners. Some, it seems, have not coped – or not wanted to cope – at all. They've felt unable to continue the relationship, have wanted to escape and start a new life. It's an understandable reaction.

> "Around this time I met the love of my life. I fell
> totally in love and thought he did with me. But by
> then I was self-medicating with booze and painkillers.
> I'd spend hours trying to read one paragraph in the
> newspaper. He soon could not cope with me – why
> should he? – and left. Part of me left too."
> *Amber, 48, oligodendroglioma Grade II/III*

> "My wife walked out when I was diagnosed. In
> hindsight, maybe she was going anyway. But I would
> not do to my worst enemy what she did: walk away
> and provide no support after 16 years of marriage."
> *Patient, oligodendroglioma Grade II*

In one very sad testimony I read, a woman knew she was falling in love with a new partner, but was considering cutting off the relationship because she knew her brain tumour would only cause long-term heartache for him and any children they might have. Getting out now would be less painful.

Other partners have taken an 'I don't want to know' approach. They're there for emotional support for the person living low grade, but don't want to get into the technicalities. They don't want to know the type of tumour, the life expectancy, the struggle that might be on the horizon. I guess they're either trying to ignore the issue, or have decided to take everything step-by-step, tackling each problem as it comes. They provide loving emotional support when it is needed, and try not to worry too much about the future.

In some rare cases, I've known this dynamic turned on its head. The brain tumour patient has not wanted to know the technicalities: they don't want to see the scans, they don't want to know about prognosis, they'll take treatment as it's offered but don't want to know why. Meanwhile, their partner has taken all this information on themselves and somehow has to deal with it alone. They've had to shield their loved one from news, whether good or bad. This burden of knowing, while the patient does not, must be unbearable. But of course it is done out of love and respect for their wishes. A very brave approach indeed.

In my own case, it took about two or three hours after diagnosis for my wife to announce something along the lines of: 'This is not *your* brain tumour, this is *our* brain tumour.' It affects both of us, albeit in different ways, was her message. We both needed to support each other. She meant it in an emotional way, of course, but also in a practical one. Making appointments, monitoring drugs, taking time off work to accommodate the condition or to care for our children was something we would work out together. It was not something she was willing to allow me to do alone. It helped me to see the immense impact that my diagnosis had on my whole family, and helped to distract me from feeling sorry for myself. Her feelings were just as important as mine, her fears just as deep. She too needed to be distracted by the practical implications, the busyness that my tumour brought. If not, she would be left to deal with the emotional side alone.

At the beginning, I seriously asked myself the question: 'Would it be better if I just disappeared? Walked away from my marriage and my kids, to spare them the pain of dealing with the condition as it progressed? Why not free my partner from the emotional and practical burden? Wouldn't that be the loving thing to do?' But I soon came to the understanding that living low grade was something my whole family was already doing, and by making myself disappear I could not prevent their distress. They would still have to deal with my disappearance and loss, or deal with never knowing what had happened to me. It would be a pain that would last the rest of their lives.

After diagnosis, whatever happened, there could be no turning back the clock. Instead, I began to fully understand what my wife was saying. We needed each other. Our children needed us, and we both needed them. Whatever life threw at us, we would deal with it together. For us, that's what being a family meant.

> "I use 'we' to talk about the brain tumour journey, because it is something my wife and I have been through together."
> *Duncan, 33, astrocytoma Grade II*

Being single

Of course, there are many low grade patients who don't have

partners, and for them there are some very similar and some very different challenges to contend with.

First is the challenge of dealing with the diagnosis alone, or at least without someone close who you see most days and with whom you can share some of the burden. It can be lonely out there without a partner, and I imagine doubly so when you're dealing with a newly-diagnosed brain tumour.

I'm not at all saying that having a partner is better than not having one. What I am saying is that dealing with things relatively alone must be very tough indeed, even totally disabling in some cases. Of course, there might be some patients who prefer to take the diagnosis upon their shoulders only. They might feel lucky not to have to impose the burden upon someone they love.

But aside from the purely emotional, there are practical things about being single and – if you want want to do so – meeting a potential new partner. When, for example, do you tell them you have a life-limiting disease? On the first date? When you've got to know each other better? When you move in together? Not at all?

There must always be the fear – and certainly not unjustified – that a potential partner might run a mile knowing the implications of the diagnosis. That it will at least bring stress and difficulties, either ongoing or eventually. That it might result in their having to care for you at some point. Or indeed, that it might end in bereavement. Add to those implications the potential – where desired – of having or adopting children and the dilemma for both the patient and the new partner must be unbearable.

> "I haven't thought too much about the implications of my tumour for any partner – after all, at the moment I do manage to live quite a full life. If I dated someone who had a problem with it, then I guess that they just

wouldn't be the right person for me. I wouldn't intentionally hide it from them, but at the same time you don't walk up to someone and say: 'Hi, I'm Angela and I've got a benign brain tumour.' You have to find the right point to tell someone."
Angela, 24, pilocytic astrocytoma Grade I

They say love will always win out in the end, but I'm not so sure. Some single people may completely lose confidence that they will find anyone even willing to continue a relationship on those terms. Others may simply make the decision to not even try, unwilling to potentially inflict the tumour on another that they may come to love. I wish there was a solution to this conundrum. Friends and family will certainly offer their invited and uninvited, appreciated and unappreciated, wisdom!

What can be concluded is that this dilemma offers further evidence that living with a low grade glioma is far from merely having an unwanted lump in our heads. The implications of the tumour are far more wide-reaching. In all matters relating to family, relationships, being single, children and similar emotional issues, this is where charities and support networks can be vital. We're not going to get that stuff from doctors, that's for sure. We're not the first to go through this stuff, and we won't be the last. Sharing, mutual support and understanding, for most people, can ease the difficulties. And they can provide tentative solutions to even the most seemingly impossible conundrums.

Telling children

Whatever the age of your children – if you have them – telling them about your brain tumour is likely to be one of the most difficult things you will ever have to do. Indeed, for some, their low grade brain tumour and its long-term implications is something parents have tried to hide from those they love the most. With low grade gliomas, which tend to have a longer life expectancy than higher grade ones, this approach is quite understandable.

Perhaps the tumour won't turn malignant until we are already long into our old age. Our children may already be adults or may, by that time, have become fully grown with their own families. The eventual death of their parents is something our adult children may already have considered or which may at least have hovered in the background as we've grown older. Why not postpone information about our deaths, if there's a chance we might die from 'old age' first? Most, I imagine, do tell their children. Particularly if their children are adults. Like anyone we love, adult children can provide love and support for us, while we in turn can provide love and support to them.

But what if your children are younger? Most low grade brain tumour patients are in their 30s and 40s when they are first diagnosed, and that means many are likely to have children who are still young, even infants. I have two children, but they were both still very young when I was diagnosed: aged two and four. They were certainly too young to have the *sit down, we've got something to tell you* conversation and wouldn't have understood what we were talking about if we'd tried.

Instead, my wife and I decided that we would let our children know about my illness by osmosis. We'd allow them to come to understand it at their own pace as they grew up. We wouldn't hide the disease from them, we'd simply carry on as a family and allow them to gradually build up knowledge about my condition. We'd talk about my tumour and cancer at home. We wouldn't hide that I had seizures or bad days when I couldn't get out of bed. They got used to the idea that I had frequent doctor's appointments and had to go into hospital every now and again.

As they got a bit older, they came to know that I was poorly and that it was something to do with my brain. They understood that doctors had opened up my head to take a look inside. As well as generally not hiding my condition from our children, we also consciously dropped it into conversation. We've talked about cancer and brain tumours, and death and that sometimes people get so poorly that they die.

At the time of writing, coming up to two years from diagnosis, I believe that my children understand that I am poorly and that I will never get better. They know I have a disease called cancer, and that mine is in my brain. They know I have seizures, and have seen me have what they call *dizzies* many times. They know I can't drive because of them. But I think they only have a peripheral understanding that it is likely to lead to my dying sometime. I'm not sure they've contemplated the idea that a mummy or daddy *can* die, though animals, distant relatives and people on the news certainly can.

But as many of us know, our children can surprise us with their perceptiveness. We've never explicitly stated that I have cancer to our children, yet my five-year-old daughter has told me that I have it. She says she wants to look after me when she grows up. She says she wants to take away the badness in my brain, and fill my head with strawberries. It breaks my heart.

I can only speak for our experience, but I know we have taken the right approach with our children. With the gradual drip-drip-drip of information, it has simply become part of their normal lives. It's not something for them to be afraid of or shocked by. They have never really known it any other way. One of the main reasons we took this approach was to avoid the shock of them finding out something terrible by accident from someone else, and becoming afraid and perhaps even emotionally scarred in the long term. We knew that at school, or among friends and family, something might be said to our children about my condition. We would rather that knowledge came to them slowly, at their and our own pace, in an atmosphere of love and safety.

We know that one day our children will each come to the realisation for themselves that Daddy may not be around forever. Those will be difficult and painful days for us all. But we hope they will be eased by an understanding of my illness that they have grown into, rather than one that has been thrust upon them suddenly. We expect to need to call on professional help at some point. Our local hospice uses figures and dolls houses, creative drawing and play to help children understand and deal with death. If they are still young when we need to get into the detail, we'll use that approach. In the meantime, the hospice has said that what we've done is sensitive and appropriate, and in their opinion right for our family and the age of our children.

> "I had nine-hour surgery, but it isn't completely cured
> and I'm told it will grow back. We told my two-year-
> old that Mummy had to go have some bad bits cut out
> of her head. She accepted it straight away. She used
> to tell people mummy has a zip in her head, because I
> had 37 staples."
> *Lindsey, 35, meningioma Grade I*

Families and loss

Can you envisage family life without you involved? That's what many low grade patients find themselves facing when they are first diagnosed. You may be very young yourself and have parents, grandparents and even great grandparents who are still alive. You may be older and have children and grandchildren. Or you may be somewhere in the middle – as I am – with children as well as parents who are still alive.

The idea of your family having to cope with your disease, and perhaps even having to carry on without you in the future, can be absolutely heartbreaking. And if it's tough for you, it's tough too for your parents and children: how do you or they even go about dealing with such an uncertain future?

In the few hours following my diagnosis my thoughts turned immediately to my family. How would they cope without me? Would my children even remember who I was? Would my wife have to care for me if I started a physical and mental decline? How would she cope after my death? As I grew to know more about low grade gliomas, there became yet further layers: I realised my wife and children were already having to deal with my mood swings, my tiredness, my seizures and other side effects. They also had to live with the uncertainty that my diagnosis brought the whole family.

> "When we first got the call to say she was in hospital in Florida we were shell shocked and panicking. We spent the next week worrying until she was safely home. From then on, at every stage, we were constantly worrying.
>
> "We have to stay strong in front of Nanette and do our crying alone. Her psychologist said it was OK to cry in front of her, but he doesn't know her as we do. We have become very protective and find it very difficult to step back and let her get on with things. I have found in the past that letting her get on with things herself doesn't always work out."
> *Jen, mother of Nanette, 38, oligodendroglioma Grade II*

As well as thinking about my family and their loss, I'll admit to some initially selfish feelings after diagnosis. I started to think about how I may not live to see my still very young children grow up. I might not see them start secondary school, and if I did, I might not see them go to university. I might miss their weddings or meeting any long-term partner. I would, essentially, miss their life: the teenage years, the tantrums, the pride, the love, the arguments, the trials and tribulations of having kids. And it broke my heart. It hurt so much that I realised these thoughts could be crippling.

First, I learned to put such thoughts out of my head. The nature of low grade gliomas is such that I might well not miss these events. I could still be around a long time into the future. But at the same time, I realised that in these questions there were demons I just didn't want to confront. We all have our weak spots, and thinking about my children growing up and my missing out on their doing so is one of mine. It may not be healthy, but it works for me to try not to think about these things. If I did, I feel like I might get tied up in knots of stress and anguish. I might not even be able to function. I could allow these thoughts to control my life, or I could try to put them out of my mind.

They're one of the only cases where I've not been happy to talk too much about my diagnosis and its long-term prospects. In this approach, for now at least, I feel comfortable.

> "I think about death a lot, I am not morbid and stay positive but I do think about it in terms of leaving my children, not watching them grow up, graduate, get married, have kids, be a success in life. This is something I have slowly got my head around but I feel cheated. I feel guilty for cheating my children. Mums are supposed to be there for life and I won't be. I never let a day go by without telling them I love them. For every achievement they make I bask in it and tell

them how amazing they are. They are the main
reason I won't go down without a fight."
Marie, 35, astrocytoma Grade II

The second strategy I've used is to concentrate – probably
a lot more than I did before – on exactly what my children are
like now. I probably appreciate them more at the age and
stage they are at, and don't wish they were any older or
moving on to the next stage. All parents love our kids for who
they are now, but also for what they're going to be in the
future. For me, the emphasis has slightly shifted to the former.
I've concentrated with wonder on every little step they make,
everything they learn, what makes them happy and how they
have already developed, and much less on what may or may
not happen at a later date. As my condition progresses, I don't
know if these strategies will continue to work for me. But right
now, they feel about right.

In the same way, I began with selfish emotions about my
wife. What would her life be like without me? Would she meet
someone else? Would she share intimacies that I once thought
would be ours alone? Would someone else move into our
house or try to be a father to my children? I realised these
were really jealous thoughts, rather than helpful ones. And as
soon I realised that, they eased and then went away entirely.
Like for my children, I realised the most important thing was
to express my love for my life partner now. Part of that would
be to accept and acknowledge that even without me, her life
will have to go on. Wouldn't I want her to have the most
happiness she could possibly have?

I worried, and continue to worry, about her life once I
have gone: but that's now about whether she'll be financially
secure, happy and safe, and how she'll cope with grief and if
she'll have the support she needs. Every now and again, I've
joked about her finding a new man when I've gone, or how

she'll have to do all the housework when I'm not around. We laugh about these things together, but we don't flog them. While I'm still low grade and pretty healthy I've decided to leave it at that. I know if and when my life becomes in danger or my condition begins to decline, we will talk about practical things we can do together to help her and the children into the future. Things around finances and support networks, about leaving good memories of me that don't feel restrictive or distressing. My wife has taken to filming me more often, to save images of my being a good dad to my children. While I often find this quite intrusive, I understand her need to do it – for herself and for the children.

It's tempting to rush into planning for every eventuality. For some, that can even be a coping strategy. But once I'd learned more about my condition, I realised there was no real rush. That things could be left until later, or done in a more laid back and reasonable way. To some extent, I've decided to procrastinate on the boring stuff, in favour of living my life while I'm still healthy. But always at the back of my mind, and sometimes on paper too, I'm creating a list of things we'll need to tackle together sometime in the future.

Finding out who your friends are

"I have to admit," said a good friend about three weeks after my brain tumour diagnosis, "I was more nervous to see you than I've ever been nervous about anything."

The interesting thing was, I'd felt exactly the same about seeing him. For both of us, we just didn't know what to say. What questions to ask. How much I wanted to tell or how much he would want to know. Of course, we quickly reverted to our usual habit: we went to a pub for a little social lubrication and were soon joking about the lump in my brain as if we were talking about sport or politics. That he'd told me about his nervousness about meeting me showed what a good friend this guy was. We've known each other since we were teenagers, and have always had an easy going and close relationship.

Learning someone you know well or even love has a brain tumour or incurable disease does change your relationship with them. It's an old cliché to say that terrible news reveals who your friends really are. I think it's a little more nuanced than that. Some friends say: 'Anything I can do?' And they mean it from the bottom of their heart. Others say it because it's the right thing to do, then they get on with their lives. It's sad to admit even some of my immediate family fell into the second group, rather the first.

But I'm hesitant to judge anyone's reaction. The responses have been as diverse as my friends, some expected while others have taken me by surprise. Some acquaintances I didn't even know well came out of the blue and became solid support, while some great friends ran for the hills. That's cool. People have busy lives, their own priorities and some people are just better at confronting difficult issues than others. No-one is to blame for their reaction. That's what relationships and personalities are all about, and I wouldn't want it any other way.

Yet, I've recognised some patterns that have chimed with other people who have long-term illnesses. I must emphasise that I classify them here not in particular judgement, but simply through convenience. Some friends and family cross these categories or end up a combination of some of them, some of the time.

Ignorers

These are the everyday friends and people who you don't necessarily know well, who hear your news for the first time and perhaps send a card or a sympathetic email telling you to let them know if there's anything they can do. Then you don't hear from them again.

Happy surprisers

These are the friends you wouldn't necessarily have called best buddies, but who then knock you over with their sympathetic, practical and emotional support. Perhaps they've been affected by cancer themselves or just naturally respond well. They come out of the blue with their generosity and understanding and you become very fond of them. It's like discovering new friends all over again.

Rocks

Usually already good friends, these are the guys who simply *get it*. They're there for you, frequently on the phone, checking in with you but knowing when to give you space too. They understand that it's not just you, but your family and your other friends too who are affected. These are the guys you can call up in the middle of the night. When they turn up to your house to see you, they bring a cake and don't expect to be treated like guests. Not because they think you're incapable, but because they know spending time with you is the priority, not cooking and washing up.

These are the guys who come to your bedside when you're about to go into surgery, and who stay with your partner while you're under the knife. They're still there when you come round again. They're the ones who visit you in hospital and pass out news to others so you're not bombarded with phone calls.

> "Laura came with me and sat with me while I waited for scans. She missed tutorials the next day, and brought me clothes and things I needed at four in the morning. I don't know what I would have done

without my two flatmates, and my other uni friends who came to visit me in hospital. They all rallied around so much to visit me on the other side of town."
Angela, 24, pilocytic astrocytoma Grade I

Sad surprisers

There will be some friends who you truly believed were some of your closest buddies, but who either can't deal with your diagnosis or appear to be unmoved. They don't call, they don't ask how you are. You don't get the feeling they're there for you and some don't even mention your diagnosis. I know some of these guys just don't want to confront an uncomfortable truth or think I don't want to discuss it, so I'm not too hard on them.

> "Someone I used to know stopped talking to me the day I came out of hospital from my second operation. I tried every method of contact, but was ignored. Then I bumped into them in a car park a few days after I had started radiotherapy. All they did was look at the floor as I spoke and since then have not made contact. I would love to get back in contact as I treasured that friendship so much."
> *Rachel, 26, neurocytoma Grade III*

Doers

These are the amazing friends – some of whom you will barely know and even their friends who you don't know at all – who do something practical to support one of the brain tumour or cancer charities. They organise a cake sale at work, run a race, cycle long miles or do a sponsored walk, because they want to *do something*. I have been consistently moved and impressed by their sheer generosity. Where possible, I have turned up and even participated in events to support their efforts. The doers have meant an awful lot to me.

Long lost buddies

Some of these are welcome, some not so much. Following my diagnosis I heard from people who'd not contacted me (and I hadn't contacted them) for more than 20 years. Some had their own stories to share, others saw an opportunity (as I did) to rekindle an old friendship. But with others, I felt an unhelpful pressure to meet up, perhaps travel half-way across the country to spend the weekend. It was all meant in good faith. But I have to admit the onrush of old friends who were suddenly interested brought with it a certain burden. After a while, I began to only connect with those I genuinely remembered fondly and wanted to get back in touch with. Selfish perhaps, but there is only so much time and emotion to go around.

Gossipers

There was one woman in my broader circle of association. She'd never spoken to me in the two years I knew her and I'd not spoken to her. For one reason or another she heard about my diagnosis and suddenly started getting very chatty. Not about brain tumours, but loads of other stuff. She treated me as if we'd been best buddies for years. I'm afraid I couldn't help feeling like I was simply the latest voyeuristic news story for her, and that my life would soon be doing the rounds among her other acquaintances.

What can I do to help?

In almost every card and email I was sent when I started telling people about tumour, I received an offer of help or the question of what they could do. To start with, I didn't know.

My family and I were still raw from the diagnosis, in a haze of grief and confusion. Just the offers and questions about doing something sustained us. They reminded us there were people out there holding us in their thoughts. Many others kept offering, desperate to help in their own little way.

Given time, and once we came to realise there was nothing our friends could actually do about the tumour or even its side effects, there were a few things we could ask from those who wanted to help. We asked people to do childcare when I had appointments. If they were mathematically minded, I asked for help to understand my finances. One friend I asked to be witness to my will, while another agreed to be its executor.

We asked for people's company, simply to be with us, which was freely given even if it meant cancelling something they already had planned. We asked for people to do something to raise money for brain tumour research, a thing that many friends and family took up with gusto. Others took on these things without even being asked. It did lead to a strange guilty feeling that people were doing these things *for me* and that I needed to be endlessly grateful. But their reaction was always that it was satisfying and rewarding to be able to make some kind of contribution.

And when none of these options were possible, I simply took to saying: 'Don't worry, when things do turn ugly my wife, my children and I will need all the support and offers of help we can get.'

The Brain Tumour Charity has created a fact sheet for friends and family who ask brain tumour patients: 'What can I do?' The ideas range from bringing food round, to offering to take the kids while you sleep or have a hospital appointment, to passing out information to others, to fundraising on behalf of the charity. There are a few books on the subject too, because friends really don't know what they can do to help.

Over time, I came to realise that our friends were not just trying to be helpful when they offered support. They were also channelling their own grief, their own feelings of impotence. While it's hard to look outwards, I had to remember that others needed their own support about my diagnosis too.

The brain tumour community

Apart from friends and family, one of the strongest sources of support I've had is from what could loosely be called 'the brain tumour community'. These are the charities, clinicians and support groups, as well as others with brain tumours, who have knowledge and experience to share. I was reticent, at first, to get in touch with a charity. I didn't want to become simply a fundraising case study (having been in charity communications for most of my working life). But when I did, I found understanding and genuine empathy with what we were going through.

A few medical staff have stuck in my mind as particularly knowledgeable and helpful, while others have been less so. Suffice to say, it was the supportive ones I kept going back to and to whom I offered any assistance I could to help their work.

But the most overwhelming support I received was from others with brain tumours. Through my blog and other associations I met low graders and others with whom I could share experiences. A few individuals read particular blogs and reached out to say they'd had the same experience, or to reassure me about things I was worried about.

I even arranged to meet up with a few. One guy I nervously met at a London train station intending to have a quick coffee; I didn't want to take up too much of his time but just say thanks for his emails. Hours later, we had had lunch and were still chatting when it was me who had to say goodbye because my train was about to leave. We shared so many experiences and reactions to our similar diagnoses, it was probably the most useful support I had from someone involved with brain tumours. All given generously and without expectation.

I pledged to myself then that where I could I would attempt to offer the same support to others. I hope this little book fulfils at least some of that pledge.

> "Tyler has done radio, video and newspaper articles. So few children are diagnosed he wanted to promote awareness of the symptoms of tumours. He is very practical and positive when doing these interviews and it really helps him as well. He doesn't really like to talk about his illness apart from when he thinks he might be able to help someone else. The charity work has given both Tyler and I something to concentrate on and helps take away some of the anger and downs that you naturally go through."
>
> *Janice, mother of Tyler, 16, glioneuronal tumour Grade I*

Feeling like a fraud

Of all the emotions I expected to go through after diagnosis with a brain tumour, I'd never marked guilt down as one that I would feel. After all, it was me with the life-limiting disease wasn't it?

In the heat of diagnosis, when I'd first heard the words brain tumour and shut off my ears to what my surgeon was telling me about the nature of low grade brain tumours, I simply thought I was going to die. And this was the general impression I gave to my friends and family. My clumsy reading of the statistics showed that I'd probably live about five to eight years, and it would be pretty much down hill from today onwards. Friends naturally showed amazing sympathy. They were generous with their time, emotion and we received piles of cards and sympathetic messages. For a short time, my family and I became the centre of people's worlds, bringing home to them the vulnerability of life. They too, or worse their children, could be affected by a terminal disease.

And then what happened? I didn't die.

Like me, my friends and family had expected the worst from my brain tumour. In some ways, we'd all prepared for my decline. We all gushed with emotion until we were spent, and then there I was still knocking around a year or more later, cycling and going for meals out as if very little had happened. And so I felt guilty and I felt like a fraud. It was as if I'd pulled off a con trick, reaped the rewards, then carried on as if nothing had changed. And this feeling of guilt kept revisiting me every time I saw friends I hadn't seen for a while. Last time they'd seen me, I was supposedly at death's door. Yet here I was, still alive and maybe even looking healthier than I did.

Like all things with low graders, this feeling of being a fraud was something I felt acutely at the start, then got used to and then it stopped altogether. One of the reasons it stopped being a problem was because things *were* actually happening and changing. It was just things I hadn't expected.

My seizures kept changing in frequency and intensity, bringing with them new dilemmas and disappointments. I constantly had to change my medication. My drugs stopped me from drinking alcohol and I'd have periods of extreme tiredness. I got depressed, then felt better again, then got depressed again. I'd constantly change my mind about what I wanted to do with my life, particularly my working life.

Then there was the change in the blood take up of my tumour. That led to my having a biopsy and another flurry of concern and sympathy from friends. And, of course, the MRI scans continued, each time bringing with them expectation, worry and then sometimes uncertain results. So I did still have a brain tumour, and all of these things were part of what, for me, is meant by having one. OK, they weren't a *decline* as such, they weren't intensive treatment and they certainly weren't death. But they were, and still are, something my family and I were going through every day. There was no fraud, and there was no reason to feel guilty.

> "Most people, including me, know very little about brain tumours until it affects them. People do not realise they cause seizures, tiredness and stroke-type symptoms. In fact I probably look normal to most and this is part of the burden."
> *Rory, 41, oligodendroglioma Grade II*

I realise in hindsight that my feelings of guilt were normal. And of course they weren't reflected in what my friends were actually thinking. They were simply glad I was still around. They hadn't forgotten about my diagnosis, and they weren't somehow wishing I'd either *get on with it* or that I'd never mentioned it in the first place.

Like all of us, they were just getting on with their lives. When we did get together, they were curious and sympathetic to hear the latest developments. And they did realise that my diagnosis affected me and my family every single day, even if I wasn't yet careering towards death. None of us can live in panic all the time. Just as I'd had to adapt my life to accommodate my low grade glioma status, they too had done the same. As my diagnosis changed, their understanding and expectations changed right along with it.

It helped that I began a blog about my condition, which many of my friends subscribed to. It described in detail the changes in my emotional and physical life, as well as giving them a heads-up for the next MRI scan or signalling any significant change any of us should be worried about. In fact, visiting friends began to joke that they didn't even need to ask how I was; they'd already checked the internet before they left home.

Guilt about our 'luck'

The other issue around guilt is that having a low grade glioma does put us in the 'better end of the bad ones' when it comes to brain tumours. And different low grades have better prognosis than others. I've sometimes felt incredibly guilty that my 'luck' meant I wasn't immediately ill, while other brain tumour patients may have lasted only a year or even months. Why should I be feeling OK, when that woman with a new baby has been given 12 months to live? How can I go out on my bike, with my relatively stable brain tumour, when that five-year-old girl is having debilitating chemotherapy that can only extend her life for a few more months and has no chance of curing her?

> "I did get better. What's left with me for the rest of my life is how much worse it could easily have been. I hear of similar stories of tumours causing haemorrhages and I don't think I've heard of any yet where anyone's gotten off with it as lightly as me."
> *Angela, 24, pilocytic astrocytoma Grade I*

> "I thought why do I get to survive yet my husband [who died from a brain tumour months before my diagnosis] didn't. I know my tumour can never become malignant from what I've been told. How is that fair? As I'd done so much research with my husband it did help knowing a lot more about tumours. But it also scared me. I knew the worst case

scenario and had to make myself accept that my journey would be completely different to my husband's."
Nicola, 35, acoustic neuroma Grade I

"When I really struggled was at the hospital when I knew that some kids were really, really poorly with such high grades that their prognosis was horrible. I knew of course that a low grade can turn into a high grade, but it was when people heard 'low grade' or 'benign'. I could see the look on their faces as if to say: 'You are so lucky.' When I've got chatting to other parents and realised that their children were not going to make it, I very rarely let on about it being low grade. It was better to say nothing at all."
Penny, mother of Harry, 17, juvenile pilocytic astrocytoma Grade I

This is the normal grief and guilt we all feel in our day-to-day lives – walking past homeless people, seeing starvation and war on the TV – but writ large because the comparisons are so much more direct. My one concrete response has been to be as helpful as I can to brain tumour and other cancer charities. It may not be much, but it is something. That doesn't mean donating all my life savings. It means offering the skills I have developed over the years in my career as a writer and trainer, using them to assist charities to be more effective and to get information out there.

If my professionally learned skills can help the charity be more efficient, get more fundraising income or raise the profile of brain tumours, then that's perhaps better than a big cheque. But I'm not naive enough to imagine that this is all a selfless act. It does also serve to assuage some of my guilt of being one of the lucky ones.

And it also reminds me that if I feel guilty about my brain tumour, how guilty my friends and family must feel for being healthy and going about their normal lives. It helps me to understand their reactions better. Ultimately, it reminds me that it's OK to feel guilty now and again. That's what being human can sometimes be about.

5

Getting medical

THOUGH IT CAN sometimes feel like you're in this alone, low grade tumour patients will accumulate a team of medical experts and others who will one way or another be involved in your life. From knowing very little about cancer at all – I'd barely even heard of the term 'oncology' before my diagnosis – I found I had to learn very quickly about the different medical experts involved in my care.

I came to understand that while I might only see one particular consultant for meeting after meeting, there was actually a whole team of people behind the scenes who would discuss my case, advise each other and make recommendations about what we should do next. It wasn't until I saw a television programme about brain tumours and a section where about a dozen people, including some junior and trainee doctors, were sitting in a lecture theatre looking at someone's MRI scans, that I understood properly the role of the multi-disciplinary team (known as the MDT).

I realised later that I would come into contact with most members of my MDT as the disease changed and progressed, but not all of them. The MDT includes both people I would meet, but also their colleagues. They check each other's work, challenge each other's decisions and work together to improve general and individual care of patients. Granted, some hospitals in the UK aren't quite so organised. But my own experience has been that the major brain tumour centres around me, in London and in Cambridge, put an effective MDT at the heart of their work with patients. That's pretty reassuring.

> "The NHS were brilliant and almost constantly charming. They have their faults, but at Queen Square for my biopsy I felt I had won the postcode lottery. I never actually met my surgeon, but the consultant and his understudy explained all the details of my tumour and how they would approach it. In the end they didn't feel surgery was appropriate and they just did a biopsy. After months of tests and appointments I realised I probably would have paid something like £70,000 for the same treatment in the United States and here I got it all for free with a smile."
> *Ben, 37, oligodendroglioma Grade II*

Your team

It is worth highlighting the key figures low grade glioma patients are likely to encounter, some of whom are key players in MDTs.

General practitioner (GP)
It was probably your GP to whom you first reported any

problems, unless your tumour was found as an accident or in an emergency. Day-to-day, low graders will see their GP only to get drugs prescriptions and sick letters signed, perhaps for the occasional check-up and to help deal with side effects of the tumour or its treatment.

GPs are generally copied into all the major letters and emails various consultants send to each other. In an ideal world, they'll know what's going on with your tumour at any one time. But they often don't, and you'll probably keep them more up-to-date than your specialists will.

Neurologist

This brain doctor will most likely be a specialist in brain tumours and possibly epilepsy too. It'll be your neurologist who you're likely to see most regularly, probably following each MRI scan. They'll probably be in charge of your drug doses, reporting good and bad news, and making specialist referrals to a brain surgeon or oncologist when some intervention is needed.

Oncologist

This is a cancer doctor, an expert in the disease and its treatment. They're usually specialists in a particular field too, so we should expect ours to have lots of experience treating brain tumours. They'll advise on non-surgical treatments, such as radiotherapy and chemotherapy, guide you through the regimes, monitor results and make changes accordingly. They'll also administer prescriptions for nausea drugs (called anti-emetics), painkillers and any other medicines.

Surgeon/neurosurgeon

Though you may not meet a brain surgeon unless you need to have a biopsy or surgery to reduce the size of your tumour, they're likely to be part of your MDT. Ahead of surgery, you're likely to discuss with them what operation they'd like to do, how they'll go about it, and of course they and their team will be the ones getting inside your skull on the day. A good brain surgeon will also follow up, checking in the next day and possibly at future meetings to discuss how the surgery went and to learn of any problems you've had.

Registrar

A registrar is a qualified doctor who is studying and specialising in a particular aspect of medicine over five to 10 years. They'll be training under a very experienced consultant (surgeon, oncologist, neurologist). They see patients alongside the consultant, or sometimes in place of them.

Clinical Nurse Specialist (CNS)

Most cancer doctors and many neurologists have a CNS working directly with them. They take much of the pastoral, support and some administrative work out of the consultant's hands, and are likely to be in more regular contact with you. It's them you're likely to first approach if your symptoms change, if you're worried about an aspect of your treatment, or if you need to arrange or rearrange appointments. The importance and support of a good CNS cannot be underestimated.

Most are experts in brain tumours, are likely to have seen much of what you're experiencing before, and will make referrals to other services such as counselling or physiotherapy if you need it. I've been extremely lucky to have been looked after by both my oncologist's and my neurologist's CNSs at different times.

Unfortunately, some low grade brain tumour patient are not allocated one at all. As I learned at one brain tumour support day hosted by The Brain Tumour Charity, low grader gliomas aren't always considered serious enough to have regular contact with a cancer nurse. In an overstretched health service that's understandable, if unfortunate. It shows again how low graders can sometimes be considered second class brain tumour patients. It's worth noting that many CNSs are at least part-funded by cancer charities, rather than by the NHS.

Radiologist

There are two types: diagnostic and therapeutic. The basic difference is that a diagnostic radiologist will oversee imaging like MRIs, while a therapeutic one deals with radiotherapy treatment.[2] They may have a good knowledge about brain tumours, but they don't generally supply information directly to patients. They will write a report for the neurologist or oncologist, which along with the images, blood counts and other results will help them determine the next move.

You

While it can sometimes feel like your medical care is out of your control, it really isn't. Except in very special circumstances, doctors and surgeons can't make us undergo any intervention without our consent. What's often missing is that the patient doesn't properly understand what's being offered to them and so offers their consent blindly.

MRI scans and results

If you've been diagnosed with a low grade tumour, chances are you're already familiar with an MRI (Magnetic Resonance Imaging) scanner. Indeed, an MRI is most likely to be the way your tumour was found and given a tentative diagnosis in the first place. For low graders, MRIs becomes a central part of our life. That's not just because we have to have them frequently – likely to be every three months to start with, then six-monthly and later yearly – but more because every MRI brings with it the fear that the tumour might in some way have changed.

What MRIs are generally looking for is a significant growth of a low grade tumour, its return after surgery, an intensity in any part of it, an increase in blood uptake or a build up of blood vessels. None of these are necessarily indications of a low grade glioma turning into a higher grade one. But they can be, particularly if they're taken together. A significant growth can also be a problem even if the tumour isn't turning malignant, simply because it is more likely to press on healthy parts of the brain or to increase pressure in the skull.

All of which is a way of saying, MRIs are important to low graders. They probably strike fear into most of us. But you do kind-of get used to them. In my experience, I only really get concerned about them on the day I go to hear the results. Of course, if that happens in a week when I've been having particularly intense or frequent seizures, I naturally feel more nervous. And when my tumour did start to increase its blood vessel volume, the following MRI six months later took on a particularly important significance.

But I've learned to take MRIs in my stride. A bothersome and worrying episode every six months, but only because I know that one day that MRI is going to be the start of bad news. A relatively *clear* MRI became a marker on my low grade journey, rather than the expected end of it. It was difficult to get to that place but it's hard to be worried all the time, particularly when you've had so many MRIs with sometimes uncertain results.

"It's hard to describe how you feel as you get closer to the scan date: nervous, anxious, scared doesn't really cover it. To me it felt like my whole world was on hold and that I was living on a different planet to everyone else. Results day is like no other as you sit and wait your turn. Even when you get some relief that there has been no change, it doesn't change the fact that the tumour is still there."

Janice, mother of Tyler, 16, glioneuronal tumour Grade I

MRIs – keep still!

Yeah, like that's easy for 45 minutes or more. One of the most difficult practical things about MRIs is the need to keep still for long periods of time. Anything from around seven minutes to an hour. The radiographer wants you to keep still so they can get a clear picture of your brain. Yet being told that seems to generate an uncontrollable urge to fidget. Suddenly your nose seems to need scratching or you wish you'd arranged your legs differently. After a while, you feel uncomfortable in the position you're in.

In my experience, it's just a case of holding out. I don't actually move as much as I think I'm going to. Radiographers will slip some cushions either side of your head to keep it still. I've often been surprised after what feels like a very fidgety MRI to be told I hadn't moved at all.

Radiographers may also talk to you through a loud speaker, telling you how long the next scan is or how many scans are remaining. You could receive between five and 10 separate scans with a brief pause in the noise between them. Another thing you'll notice is that you may be scanned on the same machine each time. That's because there are subtle differences between each machine and your doctors will want to discount any changes caused by those differences rather than your tumour.

MRIs – a few more pointers

Metal
You'll need to remove anything metal from your body, including piercings and jewellery. The radiographers will also get you to sign a lengthy form about whether you've had metal shards in your eyes, swallowed any coins, that kind of thing.

Dress
Most MRI departments have lockers, perhaps changing rooms too. But I've tended to just go in tracksuit bottoms and a light top, and to take my shoes off before I go in. It's less fuss than changing once you're there, and it's more comfortable during the MRI anyway.

Earplugs
You won't be able to listen to music during the scan because of the metal in headphones. Some MRI departments play music in the room, but you're at the whim of whatever tunes your radiographer prefers. MRI machines are extremely noisy – combinations of buzzes, clicks and whirrs right into your ears – so you'll be given earplugs or protectors.

Claustrophobia
You'll be delivered into a long tube, and will have a plastic mask placed very close over your face. If you're claustrophobic, it's worth talking to your doctor or radiographer beforehand. You'll be given a panic button to press should you start to worry too much, and you may even be given a sedative to keep you calm. I find closing my eyes and even trying to go into a pseudo-sleep helpful.

Injections and traces

Your consultant or radiographer may want to pull you out of the machine half-way through to inject you with a dye, called a 'contrast'. It allows them to trace the blood pathways in your brain. You won't be able to get up while they do it, and once it's done they'll roll you right back in again and continue. I find it disconcerting because I can't see them while they're doing it, though I often prefer not to watch injections anyway. But I do hate the creepy cold feeling, as the contrast works its way up my arm.

Safety

Despite what some quacks and snake oil salesmen would have you believe, MRIs cause no damage to your brain or body in the doses or at the frequency you'll receive them. (Though pregnant women are advised to declare their pregnancy to their consultant and radiographer). No negative effects have ever been proven, and your radiographer leaves the room only because they're working with X-rays every single day of their working lives. The only documented negative side effect I could find was one case where someone left a fire extinguisher in the MRI room, and magnetism caused it to fly up and injure the patient. A little lesson perhaps in ensuring your piercings and jewellery are removed, but testament too to how safe MRI scans really are.

Results day

By far the most frustrating aspect of MRIs is that doctors seem to take ages to interpret the results, and in my case it can be anything up to a month between the MRI itself and results day. I am being fitted into my busy consultant's packed schedule, but that doesn't make the waiting any easier. After all, don't the scans immediately turn up on the radiographer's screen? Why can't the doctor just look at them there and then, and give me the results right away?

For some patients, that's exactly what they do do. But for others a longer wait is more normal. That's because a radiologist actually writes a report about the MRI scan and their own observations, before passing the images to the consultant.[3] The challenge is to fill up the waiting time between MRI and results day.

> "After the scan it would be about a week or two weeks before getting the results, which feels like forever. Trying to get a good night's sleep the night before results was and still is difficult. I find the wait agonising because I am worried about what might be found and how it could affect me and those close to me. The way I cope is to try and not think about it and carry on as normal."
>
> *Rachel, 26, neurocytoma Grade III*

Since I've tended to have MRIs every six months, I've tried to stick a holiday or time off work between the scan and the results. This strategy has allowed me space to worry and discuss the 'what ifs' with my wife, but also freed me from the guilt of sometimes not being able to concentrate on work because: 'What's the point anyway if everything is about to go wrong?' Having something to do that isn't the everyday has helped distract me from the pending appointment. Taking my two kids on holiday and trying to keep them entertained brings with it both a blissfully busy mind and the reward of spending time with them. At least it's not sitting in a darkened room for two weeks, rocking backwards and forwards sick with worry. It might be what I sometimes want to do, but it won't make results day come quicker. And it's not going to change the result either.

On results day, I've only ever been able to feel nervous. I pretend to myself that I'm philosophical and accepting of whatever the doctor is about to tell me. But then I catch a little shake of my hands, a quiver in my voice or a black feeling deep down in my stomach. This could be the bad one, I think. I've found it's just a case of getting through the day as best you can. My wife and I treat ourselves to an expensive coffee and cake before we go in for the results, and try not to rush the travel in the morning so we don't end up waiting around too long.

It's the waiting that is most painful, particularly that time when you've checked in with the receptionist and are waiting for the meeting to actually take place. In my hospital, that wait has never been less than an hour and has sometimes been two hours. I've tried to write, I've tried to read. I've tried emailing and phoning people. I find myself constantly needing the toilet, and seek out the most remote one in the hospital so I take as long as possible. Nothing makes that wait more bearable. I wish it did. But then, once my name is called, fear turns to resignation. The inevitable is coming, there's nothing I can do about it. I might as well get on with it. I'm simply carried along by the tide and stop worrying altogether.

> "I've been doing results day for four years now and it never gets easier. In fact I say it gets harder. You know what to expect, the hum of the machine, the sympathetic looks on staff's faces, the anxious wait for the neurosurgeon to fill you in. You think while waiting: 'I'll just be happy if it's stable, please be stable.' Then the news is exactly that, and you think: 'Why hasn't it disappeared?! Why hasn't a miracle happened and it's gone?!'"
> *Marie, 35, astrocytoma Grade II*

"I have always been someone who likes to plan and
have always found that looking towards the future is
important. The initial three months after diagnosis,
waiting for the next MRI, were the hardest I've ever
been through. I had no idea how the next scan would
turn out. The results of the first follow up were
positive and the initial feeling was elation. It was the
first positive news in some time. Then the reality set
in. It would soon be three months and another scan."
Duncan, 33, astrocytoma Grade II

The very worst experience I've had so far after an MRI
was my first results day, three months after an earlier scan had
revealed the tumour in the first place. This would be the first
time we'd all see whether the tumour had grown. Previously,
we'd had nothing to compare it to. Not only did we have to
wait for an hour and a half for the results meeting but when
we went in, I was seen by a doctor I'd never met before. She
proceeded to talk in jargon for 10 minutes, then started asking
me how I was and what seizure activity I was having. All the
time I was thinking: 'Just give me the results!'

In the end the fact that the tumour hadn't grown just
slipped out as part of her general chit-chat, as if hearing those
words wasn't the very reason I'd come to the hospital that day.
I even had to double check with her: 'You mean, there's been
no growth?' The doctor seemed so oblivious to how important
that news would be to us. I later complained to her assistant
nurse:

"When a brain tumour patient comes to get the results
of their latest MRI, that's exactly what they want to
hear the moment they come in. They're not listening
to anything else the consultant is saying. They don't
want to tell you how they are. They don't want to hear

your jargon. They just want to know one thing: 'Is the news good or bad?'"

Another example is another MRI results meeting where my neurologist revealed my low grade glioma had an abnormally high vascularity score. Apart from explaining that vascularity was 'something to do with blood uptake', that was as much information as I got. It was only after going home that I came to learn that the very same neurologist had written scientific papers on levels of brain tumour vascularity, and how they can be used to predict a tumour's transformation from low grade to high grade. He was the expert on this stuff, but hadn't thought to share that information with me.

Some call this medical gatekeeping. If you don't want to know the detail it can prevent worry. Sometimes, though, it feels as if our clinicians are maintaining their authority by not quite telling us things we might want to know, but don't have enough information to ask about. Some medical practitioners don't seem to understand that just telling us our MRI is good or bad may not be enough for some patients. More detailed knowledge can help us to deal with and understand what's going on.

> "Harry started with an MRI every six months. For the past three years they have been yearly and his last one will be next year. If that proves to be clear, he will cease MRIs. I guess that will be a huge sigh of relief, although I would also feel safer in the knowledge that if it were to start regrowing, an MRI could catch it before it gets too large. One mum told me that she feels anxious that the 'safety net' has disappeared now that her son is not scanned anymore."
> *Penny, mother of Harry, 17, juvenile pilocytic astrocytoma Grade I*

"Over the next year, my seizures increased, as did my medication. The MRI's had become three-monthly due to this development, and in April 2012 I was referred directly to a surgeon to discuss the possibility of surgery. Since this had been mentioned at the very beginning it did not come as a shock. I think 'reality check' would be a better description, because it was something we had put to the back of our minds. Since my day-to-day life had so far been hardly affected, this was something that would have an impact. How much of an impact we're yet to know."

Duncan, 33, astrocytoma Grade II

What are doctors looking for?

So, what's so interesting about those all important MRI scans? When we go for our results meetings, what are the kinds of things that doctors are looking for that we might want to know about?

Growth

The rate of growth of low grade tumours can be an indication of how the tumour is progressing, as well as if it is transforming. Low grade gliomas grow very slowly, some just a couple of millimetres a year. Meanwhile, higher grade tumours grow significantly faster. MRIs can show this growth, so doctors will be looking at whether our tumours' size or volume has changed significantly from MRI to MRI, or following surgery. Importantly, doctors should be checking not just your tumour size compared with your last MRI, but all of your MRIs into the past. That'll give an overall picture of growth rate that a comparison between two MRIs can't deliver.

Vascularity

This indicates the volume of blood vessels in the tumour and is given a 'vascularity score'. It can only be seen on an MRI if a certain type of dye is used during the process, which the consultant has to specifically ask for. The creation of blood vessels in the body is called angiogenesis. The more blood vessels a tumour has, the more blood uptake it has. Some scientific papers have shown that increases in vascularity are a stronger predictor of malignant transformation than any other measure, except actual retrieval of malignant cells during a biopsy or surgery.

Enhancement

These are the patches of more intense appearance in the tumour, compared to its surrounding area. In short, the more intense patches become the more worried doctors might be, because it could indicate a more invasive and higher density tumour.

Symptom changes

Though not something that can be seen on an MRI, doctors will want to know about any side effect or symptom changes experienced since last time. Have seizures, headaches or fatigue become more intense? What about personality changes? My consultant asks my wife about personality changes, as she's more likely to notice them than I am.

It's worth stating that few doctors consider a change in symptoms by themselves as indicative of change in the tumour. Seizures, for example, can peak and trough continually with no actual growth or increased malignancy. While looking at symptoms as part of monitoring brain tumours, doctors ought to be also looking at ways to help you deal with side effects: a change of medication or referrals to physiotherapy, for example.

119

Being in control

Low grade living often brings with it a certain lack of control. Seizures, drugs, not being able to drive. And that can be pretty frustrating. But perhaps the most frustrating part is that doctors sometimes make decisions on our behalf, without either telling us what decision they've made and why, or even properly consulting us about how we feel about it. Like it or not, the medical establishment can sometimes be quite snotty or insensitive: we're the doctors here, you're the patient, so we know what's best.

> "When this surgery was carried out Tyler's eyesight was damaged further. When he came round his eyes were moving quite alarmingly. One doctor said that he looked like Professor Mad-Eye from the Harry Potter films. That was a little upsetting to say the least."
> *Janice, mother of Tyler, 16, glioneuronal tumour Grade I*

For me, striking a balance between listening closely to my doctors (after all they *are* the experts), but also informing myself as much as possible and making my own choices has been empowering. It's also given me a sense of control where other control in my life has ebbed away. The truth is we do actually have an enormous amount of control over our medical treatment. Too often, we just don't know what options are available to us.

> "Following the biopsy, Nanette was given the result and told to think about her options which were: remove, radiotherapy or watch and wait. But at her next appointment, she was told it had been decided to leave things for three months when a scan would be

done. Nanette commented that it was not the answer she expected. She thought she would have some say in her treatment [particularly because she was concerned about the side effects of the steroids she was taking]. We decided to complain in writing and were offered a second opinion with oncology at a local hospital. They referred Nanette back for an awake craniotomy."

Jen, mother of Nanette, 38, oligodendroglioma Grade II

"I still live in fear with my tumour, every time I get a headache I panic in case it's growing again. My neurosurgeon told me I won't have another scan until four years after surgery but I will be requesting one in my review in February as I can't carry on panicking all the time."

Nicola, 35, acoustic neuroma Grade I

In the majority of cases we can decide whether to have or refuse treatment like surgery, chemotherapy and radiotherapy. There have been some sensationalised stories in the media about judges being asked to enforce decisions made by doctors, against a brain tumour patient's (or their family's) wishes. But these are very specific and complex cases, not a general rule. In short, doctors may give their professional opinion, but the patient gets to decide. What many of us might not be clear about is what right we have to choose who our doctors are, and what information about our health we're allowed to see.

"When I was told I couldn't make a decision, there was a small part of me that was relieved. I didn't want to make the decision as emotionally I wasn't thinking straight due to my grief. On the other hand I didn't

like not being able to decide for myself. I'm generally a strong, positive person, so I told myself what will be will be. I knew my husband would be watching over me and would keep me safe. I had to put my trust in the professionals."
Nicola, 35, acoustic neuroma Grade I

Different patients want to know more about their condition than others. I'm on the 'more' side, and I've found the following strategies have been enough to give me the level of knowledge I want.

Received medical letters

Very often, consultants and surgeons write to your GP to keep them informed of your condition. Your GP's surgery will keep a central file relating to your treatment, as well as any other health issues. (The NHS doesn't seem to have caught up with the 21st century enough to actually use email to do this job). You should, as a matter of protocol, be copied into these letters. If your consultant writes to your GP to summarise a recent appointment, you should get a copy of that letter through the post too. If you're not getting those letters, you're entitled to ask for them. If they refuse, which I would imagine is rare, there are legal recourses you can take to ensure you get to see them.

Getting your medical notes

Patients have a legal right to see each and every note, and every record made by doctors about them in the NHS. This includes scribbles in a paper file to computer records. Sometimes it's a case of simply asking, and if you're lucky doctors get admin staff to make a copy there and then. Patients can also get a copy of the images taken during MRI scans, usually on a DVD.

"My neurologist talked me through it all and gave me the scan CD to pass on to other doctors. I was actually allowed to take it home and could track back and forth like a movie through the slices of my brain. It was amazing."
Ben, 37, oligodendroglioma Grade II

Sometimes doctors may be more resistant (often due to the bore of administration, I imagine) and more formal procedures have to be used to get the information we want. In those cases, an application can be made to see medical records under the Data Protection Act. That entails writing to your doctor, GP or hospital with a Subject Access Request (SAR). You don't have to give a reason.

The more detailed you are about your records ('I'd like records made during my hospital stay from 14 January to 18 January on the Sunrise Ward') the better, simply due to tracking down your paperwork. You can see any health records for free (at the surgery or hospital) if they've been updated in the last 40 days. If they're older, you may have to pay up to £10 and the same if you want an actual copy of the records. Best practice suggest hospitals should take no more than 21 days to comply, though they have a legal maximum of 40 days. To get a copy of your MRI scans on DVD, prepare to pay a little more, not for the records themselves, but for the time it takes to burn the DVD and the cost of the DVD itself. You can download software, for free, to view the scans.

I wanted a copy of my first MRI scans and I had to jump through a number of hoops to get them. My first consultant didn't make it easy. I wrote to him under a SAR and though I knew he had copies in his system, he refused to give them to me directly. Instead, he insisted I wrote another SAR to the hospital where the MRI was actually done. The hospital initially directed me to the private company that had done the

MRI on their behalf, and they agreed to provide the scans and were very helpful. But the time they wanted to take was too long because I needed the scans to show a private consultant. In the end, a very kind receptionist in the NHS radiology department said she'd get a copy done if I was happy to pick them up the following morning. I paid £35 (the maximum charge is £50) and had to take along identification. It shouldn't have been so complex, but that's just the way the NHS works sometimes.

Getting a second opinion

Patients have a legal right to ask for a second expert opinion, though any second expert you're referred to isn't obliged to provide one. My first consultant was very happy to refer me to someone else, and though it took a little time, I was seen by another consultant at a different hospital. He may have confirmed my first surgeon's recommendations (a watch and wait policy) but I felt more reassured by his attitude than my first surgeon's. It later turned out that this new consultant ran one of the UK's leading multi-disciplinary teams on brain tumours and was involved in the frontline of brain tumour research.

Partly because I was in a rush to find out more about my condition – my first surgeon had essentially told me to go home and not worry about it – and partly because he'd been recommended by the charity brainstrust, I also paid £300 for a private consultation with a brain surgeon. He again said I'd received good advice, but he recommended I move my supervision away from my local hospital and into the care of his colleague neurologist. The neurologist was an expert on low grade gliomas at the National Hospital for Neurology and Neurosurgery in London (known as The National). It later turned out, when I did have a biopsy, that the same consultant I'd seen privately carried out the surgery, but this time on the

NHS. Many NHS surgeons and neurologists, it turns out, also have a private practice.

Changing doctors

Until suggested by him, I had no idea you had a legal right to change doctors and I was delighted to find that out, so I moved my care to The National. In the NHS, there is a legal right to change your GP and to decide which hospital is primarily responsible for your care. This was the right I exercised when I moved to The National. For me all it took was to formally ask my GP to transfer me, which he was happy to do. However, The Brain Tumour Charity reports that its support team deals with many queries and problems on this issue, so it seems very clear that other patients' experiences have been far from as straightforward as mine. Perseverance, the charity finds, usually pays off in the end.

The legal right to change doctors comes with a few exceptions, such as if you are detained under the Mental Health Act, if you're in the armed forces or are a prisoner. But that's still a matter of not having a legal right, rather than what might actually happen if you ask. Sometimes, it seems, neither patients nor doctors know of your right to change.

> "I had been transferred to a hospital and I asked them to re-scan me as treatment was not working. My sight was deteriorating and I suspected I did have a tumour. The consultant refused to have another MRI done saying he had reviewed the original scan and it was fine and I did not have a tumour. My health continued to deteriorate with sight and headache problems as well as lethargy and tiredness. Eventually, as there was no clear diagnosis of what was wrong with me, I sought a second opinion. My GP at the time refused to transfer me to another hospital. I had

to discharge myself from his care and after a long
period I was allowed to register at another GP
practice. And subsequently I had an MRI at another
hospital."
Paul, 58, meningioma low grade

It's up to us how much or how little we want to be
involved in our medical life. Some wish to put everything in
the hands of our doctors, and that may be a reassuring and
less stressful way of going about things. But my wife and I
found that being intimately involved helped us to fully
understand my condition. It also helped to give the medical
establishment a wider picture of our lives too. Doctors, for
example, are unlikely to take into account childcare needs,
your working life or hobbies when advising you. It's simply not
their job. Making clear what your non-medical priorities are
can help them balance your personal life with their medical
recommendations.

That sometimes leads to a change in what they're
planning. The trick is to speak up for yourself. And that's not
always easy to do. In the heat of the moment in a consultant's
10- or 20-minute meeting, I've sometimes found it hard to take
the initiative or occasionally even to get a word in. I've found
that doing my own research as well as consulting charities and
other doctors who aren't part of my medical team gives me a
little more power. I go into meetings with a list of questions
and points I would like to make. I then try not to leave the
room without checking each one off. The charity brainstrust
provide ready-made checklists for you to use.

6

Treatment

WHAT IS TREATMENT for? It may seem like a strange question to ask, and that's probably why some brain tumour patients don't actually ask it. But without understanding what we're actually trying to achieve by having some kind of treatment for our low grade gliomas, how can we hope to make any kind of informed decision about what we have and when we have it?

Remember, I'm not attempting to write a medical or science manual here. Instead I offer only a very general overview, with first hand experiences thrown in to give you an impression of what treatments are like.[4]

An important starting point simply has to be that for most low grade gliomas, there currently is no *cure* in the traditional sense. Treatment of any kind is not likely to make your brain tumour go away forever and completely, and nor is it going to stop lower grade brain tumours from eventually transforming into higher grade ones. That is, of course, the bad news.

But treatment can be, in principle, almost as good as a cure for some low grade glioma patients. That's because low grade tumours grow very slowly, and because the time of their transformation from low to high grade is unpredictable. It can sometimes be many many years. In short – and this is the better news – treatment can sometimes hold our tumours at bay for a very long time.

So what really is the main aim of treatment for low grade brain tumours, if they can't be cured in the traditional sense? The main aim is to remove some or all of the tumour, or to shrink it. Through surgery, radiotherapy or chemotherapy, the aim is to remove or kill off as many tumour cells as possible.

And why do that? First, if your low grade glioma is growing slowly, then taking away as much as possible means there's a *smaller* amount to grow slowly, effectively offering us more time while it grows back again. That, in turn, means the tumour is exerting less pressure in the head, so the damage caused by the growing tumour to the brain tissue is reduced, as are the side effects we experience. So effective treatment can both prolong our lives and improve its quality.

Second, the science has shown that certain treatments on certain tumours can lengthen the time until low grade gliomas turn into higher grade ones. The details and effectiveness vary considerably, depending on our own conditions, but in a very real sense treatment can sometimes prolong the time until our tumours turn malignant.

In other words, treatment of some sort – where we can have it, and where we're willing to have it – is generally considered a good thing for low grade gliomas. The questions are: what, how and when?

Having a brain biopsy

"It is likely we're going to have to intervene here at some point to obtain a histology."

This came as part of a formal letter from my consultant neurosurgeon. It basically said that while my brain tumour wasn't operable, I would at some point need a biopsy to discover exactly what kind of tumour it was. The histology (type of tumour) can dictate what kind of treatment might work best to halt its progress, as well as give doctors information about the genetic markers within the tumour. Genetic markers can help doctors see what kinds of treatments are most likely to work.

For many suspected low grade brain tumour patients, a biopsy will be on the agenda at some point. Sometimes doctors will go straight to surgery, during which a biopsy will be taken. But sometimes an early biopsy will be done first to get a tumour type down on paper.

What would happen, I was told, would be that surgeons would cut a small bore hole into my skull. Then a computer-guided needle would be stuck in to take a piece of the tumour, hopefully the area that my doctors were most worried about. There were of course risks. I could come out with some unspecified long- or short-term brain damage. For me, that might mean weakness or even paralysis on my right hand side, and speech difficulties. Basically a version of my seizures, but longer-term or even permanent. There were also, of course, the general risks of going under anaesthetic, and an overall risk of complications which meant I could die on the operating table.

I was to be put under anaesthetic and was assured that the risks were very small. So I decided to go ahead. But looking back, I realise there were a whole load of things I didn't know about my biopsy. Things I hadn't been told and things that had never occurred to me. I had done my own research, but everything I'd found was about what technically would actually happen *during* the procedure, not about the experience of having a biopsy. For that reason, I share the story of my biopsy step-by-step. If you're likely to have one, I hope it offers an impression of what happens. Much of it will also be relevant to those who have full brain surgery. I hope it at least helps patients to ask doctors and surgeons the right questions.

I had been given a date for my biopsy, and was asked to come in the day before. They would confirm by phone that I should come in the morning of that day before. The idea was that since my operation wasn't urgent, I'd be bumped to a different date if a more urgent case came in. That seemed fair enough to me, if a little unsettling to not know until the day before that I was going to have brain surgery. I did get that call and a few hours later I was being shown to my bed. A nurse came along and put a white band – with my name and hospital number – around my wrist and another around my ankle. She then took my observations: my temperature, blood pressure and pulse, recording it on a chart at the end of my bed. This was something that would be repeated every three or four hours during my stay.

Not long after arrival, a surgeon came to visit me in my bay. He explained the procedure and the risks, but missed out some of the things I was only later to learn. He checked it was the left side of my brain that would be operated on and, for good measure, drew an arrow pointing upwards on the left side of my neck using a marker pen. Then it was lights out. A stern nurse ordered me to put on some tight socks she'd supplied, to prevent deep vein thrombosis. And then she instructed me to go to sleep. From midnight I should neither eat nor drink.

But at 3am the same nurse returned to wake me up again. She attached 10 small spongy circles to various parts of my head, then coloured the centre of each one with a green marker pen. The stickers would help guide the biopsy and keep my head in the same place. Then she instructed me to go back to sleep. That I did, but only after a sneaky trip to the toilet to check out my new look.

The next morning another surgeon came to see me and explained he would be leading the biopsy. He said I should be up and running normally and able to go back to work in about five weeks. A nurse put a cannula (a needle containing a small plastic sheath) into my arm. When the needle is removed, it leaves the sheath sticking into the vein, into which various fluids and medicines can be pumped.

About 10 minutes later a porter arrived to get me. By this time, I'd put on a surgery gown and we walked together down to the surgery department. In a tiny waiting room, an anaesthetist explained that she would give me a mild anaesthetic to start with – through my cannula – and then a stronger one once I was asleep. I then signed a document indicating I understood everything I'd been told. I went with the anaesthetist to a pre-surgery room, where men and women in blue and green surgery gowns were milling around. After some small talk, my anaesthetist plunged a syringe into the cannula. And I was out.

The funny thing about going under anaesthetic is that it's nothing at all like falling asleep. You go out quickly, and then it feels like you're coming round again in a matter of seconds. There's no sense of time passing like there is when you sleep. As soon as I was out, I was back again. But I'd actually been under anaesthetic for five hours. I woke in a recovery room, staring at the ceiling. As I lay there, I went through a few rudimentary checks: I moved each of my fingers, starting with the right hand (the side we worried might be affected by the operation) and then the left. The same with the toes. I counted out loud to myself, testing my speech to see if that had been affected. To my ear at least, it hadn't been.

I must have drifted in and out of sleep, because every now and again a doctor would come over to test my reactions. He asked me to count aloud, to push against and then pull his hand; the same with my feet. Eventually I came round fully. A porter came and wheeled me up to the ward. I had a tube delivering oxygen under my nose and a huge plaster covering the front left of my head. I had two metal staples in either side above my ears, and I was attached to a drip rehydrating me.

Apart from that, well I felt just fine; I realise with hindsight I was still sky-high on drugs. Apart from being very hot and thirsty (natural side effects of the anaesthetic) and dropping off every now and again, I had nothing to complain about. My wife and friends have since told me my language was very slurred that evening, but no-one told me at the time.

The next morning I woke with a headache, but the nurses brought me paracetamol. After a hospital breakfast came a visit from the surgeon who told me everything had gone to plan. He'd taken eight microscopic pieces of the tumour and they had been sent down to the lab for analysis. I'd get my results in a few weeks time. I left the hospital mobile enough to get public transport home. After a couple of days on painkillers, with a fair bit of rest, I felt well enough to do some work and to look after the kids. Just over a week later I was back riding my bike. So much for the five weeks recovery.

But there were some things that doctors hadn't told me about the biopsy, which I do wish I'd known about in advance. As I understood it, the surgeon would drill a small coin-sized hole in my head. What he hadn't said was that he would have to cut a three-inch gash in the skin over the hole to get access. That meant a massive wound running from my forehead backwards. It took me totally by surprise, though in fact it did heal into just a small scar in the end, with a dent where they'd drilled the hole.

The surgeon had also shaved my hair around the wound, not something that particularly bothered me because I have rather little anyway. But for those with long hair, it probably is something we'd appreciate knowing in advance. I also hadn't been told about the staples in the side of my head, nor the excruciating pain my local nurse would inflict when prizing them out with tweezers. They'd been put in to close up small holes in the side of my head, where a metal frame had been screwed to keep my head still.

All in all, my biopsy felt much more worrying than it turned out to be. I was scared of the unknown, but also philosophical about what might or might not happen to me. Looking back now, it feels like it was nothing – just routine. But at the time, for my wife, my family, friends and I, it felt like a very big deal indeed.

Watch and wait

For a long time 'watch and wait' was the preferred strategy for low grade glioma patients. Particularly where the tumours are not causing significant side effects or affecting quality of life. It basically means doing no immediate treatment. Instead the patient is scanned every three, six or even 12 months to see how things go. Only when something changes might treatment be offered. Considering the risks and side effects of brain surgery, many surgeons and consultants will prefer a watch and wait strategy and only do surgery if things change.

That used to be the generally accepted strategy, but the scientific evidence is slowly indicating a change. In the last decade or so, the science has been pointing to earlier surgery for low grade gliomas. That's where surgery is possible and likely to be effective. It is then followed by other treatments either straight away, or after a subsequent period of watch and wait.

Doctors will have their own opinions in the ongoing debate, as well as being influenced by the particular size, location and everything else about any particular tumour. Unless your life is in immediate danger, they won't move to surgery lightly and certainly not if you'd prefer to hold on until you're ready. Watch and wait isn't an option to be dismissed out of hand, even if your first instinct is: 'I just want this thing out of my head now!'

Some low grade glioma patients spend many many years on watch and wait. They may have no intervention at all, or just a biopsy. They lead very normal lives, perhaps only with drugs to control seizures or headaches. Other than the regular and worrying MRI scan regime, low grade lives can be very full, very long and very enjoyable. Some days, we may even forget we have a brain tumour at all. The main problem with watch and wait is that doctors sometimes tend to forget that they only see us every six months or every year. They assume it's always easy for us to get on with our lives and forget our tumours. After all, we're not dying yet. That means watch and wait patients may not get the sympathy and understanding we might perhaps expect about our emotional health and the consequences of lives lived with uncertainty.

Surgery

"My tumour could be removed, so there was no question about going ahead. I remember saying goodbye to my four wonderful children before I went into hospital and writing a private letter to my husband. This was very emotional. The morning of the day I went in, he and I visited a favourite country spot of ours and enjoyed a lovely walk in the winter sunshine. All surgery carries some risk, and we were very aware that I might not come through this. It was very difficult saying goodbye, but I was quite calm and collected in the hospital ward and going down to theatre."

Jenny, 65, meningioma

Here's the bad news first. Some low grade gliomas simply aren't operable at all. Tumours may be wrapped around vital blood vessels; they may be intimately enmeshed with parts of the brain that are responsible for keeping you alive; they may be located in parts of the brain responsible for thinking, movement, breathing. In these circumstances – and mine is one of those – surgery just isn't going to happen. It would be too dangerous, or likely to lead to such poor quality of life afterwards that letting the tumour run its course would be preferable.

Here's a little more bad news. The science shows that a very large amount of your tumour needs to be removed by surgery for it to have a significant effect on your overall outcome. Taking away a few chunks here and there, but leaving most of it in because it's inaccessible, is not likely to prolong life or impede transformation. In those cases, doctors won't advise surgery. Given many low grade gliomas are diffuse – intimately enmeshed with the brain, rather than in one convenient round lump – achieving that surgery threshold can be a challenge.

But surgery certainly does happen frequently for low grade gliomas. Advances in brain surgery techniques are also chipping away at the problem of getting more tumour out without damaging surrounding tissues. The ironic good news is that if you are offered brain surgery, your surgeon will firmly believe it is safe for you and will probably be effective in your case. The risks to the brain itself, and to your life, will be explained in detail. But surgeons do report as high as an 80% to 90% rate of operations with no significant problems.

A craniotomy (essentially brain surgery) will involve putting you under anaesthetic, cutting away a piece of skin and opening your skull. Surgeons will perhaps cut into part of your brain to get to the tumour, and then cut the tumour away or suck it up using a vacuum tube. In some circumstances, your surgeon may want to wake you up during the brain surgery. This is so they can prod on different parts of the brain to see whether what they're doing is going to affect your speech, movement or other functions. This is called an awake craniotomy. Though it sounds horrible it is again considered quite safe and is a regular feature of brain surgery.

> "I didn't know you could do brain surgery while awake so I wanted to be knocked out. But when you are told of paralysis risks, it is an easy decision to make. The operation went to plan, though I had constant localised seizures in my left arm throughout. You get the pleasure of only getting fluid from a small sponge on a sausage stick. It is extremely tiring no matter how stubborn or fit you think you are, and towards the end it was very hard to stay awake. Although not a process I would choose to do every day, the awake craniotomy is a miracle in my eyes."
> *Rory, 41, oligodendroglioma Grade II*

Once as much of the tumour is removed as possible, your skull will be put back in place, the skin sewn back and the operation will be over. You may have a tube running into your head to start with, to drain off any fluid that swells around or into the gap left by the surgeons, but this will probably be removed after a day or two.

> "We discussed the procedure itself and then the outcomes. The aim of the operation was to remove as

much of the tumour as possible. This in turn would reduce the effect of growth, and also allow the doctors to determine exactly what form and grade the tumour was. Then we discussed the possible negative outcomes: the possible speech problems and some paralysis on the right side of the body. The chance of these problems was less than 10%.

"Prior to the operation I underwent a functional MRI and had a meeting with a neurolinguist. The MRI was similar to a standard one, only I was required to perform reflexes to determine the functionality of different parts of the brain. The neurolinguist tested my speech, general mental skills, and we also discussed my life and things I had a general interest in. This information would be used during the operation.

"I had an awake craniotomy. I was taken up to surgery and given sedatives. This put me into a deep enough sleep that I would not feel the initial part of the operation, but would allow me to be woken when required. The first thing I recall from the operation was when I woke up and could see the neurolinguist and anaesthetist. I was lying on my side with my head clamped in position and a drape hanging over my body. This meant I could only see things in my direct eye line. The surgeon spoke to me, explaining what they were doing and what each step would be.

"The first stage was mapping my brain. This involved the surgeon touching different parts around the tumour to see which senses were closest and how my body reacted. At one point my arm suddenly started moving up and down without me doing anything. As soon as they stopped touching that part, the movement stopped. Although I had been told this may happen it felt very strange to be almost totally under the control of other people. As the operation continued, I spoke constantly to the neurolinguist. It became clear after the first speech tests that this part was fine and so for the remainder of the operation we talked about my love of travel, sport and my family. The surgeon checked I was OK at all times, while the anaesthetist was keeping a close eye on me, ensuring that I had the right amount of medication to keep me awake but also to ensure no undue pain.

"In total I was awake for around 90 minutes, with the operation taking in total around four to five hours. Once I was sedated further for them to replace the section of skull that had been removed, I was able to hear the pins being tapped in. I felt no pain, but found the whole experience fascinating.

"On waking up after the surgery, it became obvious that one of the possible negative effects had happened. I had no feeling in my right leg, which meant I had to learn to walk again.

"There are some things in life we take for granted, like the ability to get from A to B on our own two feet. Having gone into the operation very optimistic, spending six weeks recovering in a rehabilitation centre was not something we had counted on. I was forced to evaluate my life, accept what had happened, but most importantly understand that I could still do many of the things I had always done."
Duncan, 33, astrocytoma Grade II

Side effects? Well, you can expect a headache for a day or two. By particular luck, though, the brain itself does not have pain receptors. Much of any pain we have will come from the entry wound and bruising. More seriously, brain surgery can inevitably have both short- and long-term effects on your movement, speech, hearing, vision, memory and other cognitive functions depending on where the tumour was. Your surgeon wouldn't have operated if the risk of long-term damage to these was significant, so there's every likelihood that things will slowly get back to relative normality. Afterwards, physiotherapy and other assistance may be offered to retrain or assist you to do anything you seem less able to do. A good result from surgery isn't always the case though. There are always going to be risks and unforeseen outcomes.

> "Tyler walked into the hospital fit and healthy; when he came out six weeks later he was in a wheelchair, much heavier due to steroids, constantly sick due to damage to his brain and he also had damaged eyesight. What has happened to his eyes is incredibly rare. Even London only sees a couple of cases a year."
> *Janice, mother of Tyler, 16, glioneuronal tumour Grade I*

The other risks of brain surgery are commensurate with other types of surgery: deep vein thrombosis, heart problems, bladder problems and risks associated with anaesthetic. Each of these will be taken into account, monitored and mitigated as part of your after care.

One almost certain outcome of having brain surgery is that you're going to end up with a pretty large and prominent scar. This in itself can lead to uncomfortable questions, low self-esteem and confidence, and basically makes you thoroughly fed up. Though scars turn out much less prominent than they used to be, the likelihood of having one that is totally inconspicuous is pretty slim. Some choose to grow their hair long to cover what they can, others might wear wigs. Others might embrace their scar, wearing it as a badge of honour of 'fighting' their tumour. Many of the cancer and brain tumour charities have specific supportive advice on dealing with hair loss and prominent scars.

> "In preparation for the operation I shaved my hair short as I knew I would have none afterwards on one side. I was in hospital for five days, but I made sure the day I came out I went to pick my children up from school – determination!"
>
> Marie, 35, astrocytoma Grade II

Chemotherapy

Chemotherapy for brain tumours is essentially the administration of drugs in a variety of ways that aim to kill off brain tumour cells and/or prevent them from dividing and spreading.

Some types of chemo will only hit brain tumour cells, but many will also affect healthy cells in the brain and elsewhere. This is why side effects of chemo can be pretty harsh: it's the healthy cells taking a battering too. But that also shows why chemotherapy side effects tend to clear up not too long after the treatment stops. The healthy cells get replaced, while the tumour cells may be knocked out for longer or killed off completely.

The drugs used in chemo, their method of delivery and the regime (length of time and frequency), are so variable and extensive they couldn't all be covered here. You should seek specialist information and guidance about your own proposed chemo regime, its effectiveness and side effects. But you're likely to be on a chemotherapy regime for a long time: many months, a year or perhaps even more. That's because the drugs need to hit brain tumour cells again and again to really stop them in their tracks. A single dose just isn't up to the job.

As a general impression, these are the main ways chemotherapy is delivered:

Intravenously
That is, through a drip or injection. You'll go to hospital, generally as an outpatient, to have it fed directly into your blood stream.

Orally
These are tablets you'll take regularly, and might be taking for anything from a couple of weeks to a whole year.

Cranial wafers
These are little slices of chemo drugs that can be placed into the cavity left after brain surgery. They gradually release the drug in the area that most needs the treatment.

Many chemotherapy regimes combine two or more of these delivery mechanisms, using different chemo drugs for ultimate effectiveness. When I have treatment, I've already been told what it will involve. I'll have chemotherapy after radiotherapy (see below) and that will involve six cycles of six weeks' treatment (lasting 36 weeks in total). At the beginning of each cycle, I'll go into hospital for an intravenous drip of one of the drugs. I'll then take other drugs orally, at home, for the following weeks. After a short break, the next cycle will begin. Throughout, my oncologist will monitor my white, red and platelet blood cells, to ensure not too many are being killed off to allow my body to function properly. They'll tweak my regime, or medication if my blood cell counts are too low.

Chemo side effects?

The most typically assumed side effect of chemotherapy tends to be hair loss. In fact, many chemo drugs for brain tumours don't result in much, if any, hair loss these days. If you do lose hair, it may come out in clumps or in various places. It's unlikely to grow back for a while afterwards. The other most frequently assumed side effect of chemo is nausea and vomiting. This is more likely than hair loss, though anti-nausea drugs have improved considerably and are likely to head off the worst of it. The other big side effect is fatigue. Your body will take a battering from chemotherapy, so especially towards the end of your treatment you're likely to become very tired indeed.

Doctors advise that both taking short regular naps, as well as very short periods of low intensity exercise, can help with fatigue and improve your energy levels. If all else fails, you may be prescribed medication to help tackle extreme fatigue.

Other side effects include mouth ulcers and weakened teeth (you may be eligible for free dental care if you have chemo), thinner blood (so difficulty with blood clotting if you cut yourself), fever or susceptibility to colds, constipation or conversely diarrhoea.

Let's not kid ourselves. Chemo is harsh. You'll be lucky if you get off without side effects. But these side effects will go away after treatment is over. Not straight away, but they will go. And chemo works. Oncologists wouldn't put us through it if it didn't make a difference in most cases.

> "Harry's regime was carboplatin (a nasty drug) through a drip every six weeks. He had to be in a bed in the day ward for half an hour, in case of immediate side effects. Then he also went every week for an injection of vincristine from an oncology nurse.

"The treatment reduced his immunity and blood counts so he had to be admitted for blood transfusions when red blood cells went too low, and be given intravenous antibiotics when he caught an infection.

"Harry was always fine during, but afterwards the sickness would set in. When the red count went down he would feel tired, was pale and didn't want to do anything but sit inside and watch TV. The worst thing was – when his blood count was very low - telling family and friends to stay away in case they brought germs in.

"But kids do bounce back and once he had more blood and antibiotics he was himself again for the last two weeks. Then the whole damn process would start again."

Penny, mother of Harry, 17, juvenile pilocytic astrocytoma Grade I

Radiotherapy

Radiotherapy may be less harsh than chemotherapy in terms of immediate side effects, but it can certainly be more inconvenient. Very often it will involve a daily trip to hospital (excepting weekends) for anything between two and six weeks. That's not too bad if you live near the hospital, but it's a real pain if you don't. And guess what? Many low grade glioma patients aren't allowed to drive, making it doubly inconvenient. If you are on benefits in the UK, you can get help with transport costs, but there's still the daily grind of actually going for the treatment itself.

"I had six weeks of five-days-a-week sessions. I came through this amazingly well: no steroids, no sickness and no head burning. But the strength you need to drag yourself out of bed every day to face the machine is out of this world. I found myself counting down in chunks of five days, and the six weeks went surprisingly quickly. The fatigue after was quite full on, but came in waves. I managed to write a first class final year dissertation in the three months afterwards, something I am immensely proud of."
Marie, 35, astrocytoma Grade II

"The hardest part of radiotherapy for me was the daily grind of travelling to and from the hospital. Some days I would be there and back in no time, while others, with traffic and delays, it would take hours. The timing of the therapy for me also made it a particularly difficult time as it fell over Christmas and New Year. Combining all of this with the main side effect of tiredness was very difficult. I tried to remain as positive as possible, my wife helped by making a 'radiotherapy advent calendar' so could see the light at the end of the tunnel. I did lose my hair about half way through, but since I had a shaved head I managed this quite easily."
Duncan, 33, astrocytoma Grade II

Radiotherapy works by very accurately zapping brain cells with high doses of radiation. It aims to kill off brain tumour cells by altering their DNA, but inevitably kills off surrounding brain tissue too which may have a few tumour cells lurking in there. The point of radiotherapy is that while your healthy brain cells can effectively *fix* their DNA, your tumour cells are much slower off the mark. Daily treatment doesn't give them time to recover, so gradually reduces the number of tumour cells.

Again, there are umpteen different forms of radiotherapy and more types of radiotherapy regimes. Recommendations, as always, will be based on particular tumour type, size, location and all the rest.

In general, though, this is what's likely to happen. You'll go into hospital for tests and to have a plastic mask moulded to the shape of your face. This is to ensure that each time you have radiotherapy, the radiation beams are guided to exactly the same place. Your mask will have marks on it, which the therapeutic radiologist will use to line up the machine. Each day you'll wear this mask as the radiotherapy takes place. It usually takes between five and 15 minutes. You should feel no immediate side effects from treatment itself. You'll probably feel just the same as when you went in.

"Radiotherapy was suggested after I had a brain haemorrhage while swimming. I could have either waited to what would happen or opt for it now. I and the specialist both agreed that it was time now, due to having a rare brain tumour and one that had previously bled.

"I had a six-week regime, attending five days a week. Prior to this I had to have all the scans to ensure that when they zapped the tumour they were hitting it as accurately as possible. At this time I was working in my army regiment's operations room, and was also working as a Physical Training Instructor within the army.

"I had to go and get my mask fitted. This day was strange, having a clay mask put over your face so that they could mould a plastic face cover later to be used during treatment. After receiving my new plastic face, the first time I was clipped to the bed was horrible. My head couldn't move. I'm not claustrophobic but I can fully understand why people with this phobia would panic. That dreaded plastic mask! I still have mine in my fancy dress box. I haven't used it yet but one day I will.

"My first session was OK, though I was a bit nervous as I didn't know what it would feel like. The first few weeks, I would return back to work after treatment in the morning. Up to weeks three and four, I was still taking the troops out on physical training, proudly sporting my bald patches. I was told I needed to rest, but I carried on. I had to.

"The reality of radiotherapy hit me when my son pulled a clump of my hair out. All I could do was laugh. It was now time to shave the hair off and now, to me, I looked ill. I avoided mirrors for a while because I hated what I saw. I am not ill, I refuse to say it. I now have all of my hair back fortunately.

"I have imagined that radiotherapy works as a net and currently the net is preventing my tumour from growing any further. This will last for five years, so I have set myself up that something could happen once that time is up. But I am stronger than it. I won't be beaten."

Dan, 28, malignant pleomorphic xanthoastrocytoma Grade II

Radiotherapy side effects?

Radiation does come with both short- and longer-term implications. In the short term you're likely to become more and more fatigued and this is likely to continue even after treatment is complete. Doctors' advice is the same as for chemo: allow yourself to rest and take short bouts of light exercise.

You may also lose a little hair and experience some mild 'sunburn' in patches where the treatment is given. You'll be given moisturiser to help with the burns and will need to stay out of the sun so as not to make it worse. You may want to use mild or baby shampoo to reduce the irritation.

The longer-term side effects of radiotherapy are considered more serious, but are rarer. Sometimes long after the treatment is finished, you might experience some tumour-like side effects that are nothing to do with the tumour at all: memory loss, seizures, hormone imbalances, fatigue and mood change.

You may also suddenly be surprised that your MRIs show patches of enhancement; what looks like more brain tumours. These can happen even many years after radiotherapy. These are actually changes in your normal brain tissue as a result of the radiotherapy called radionecrosis: essentially lumps of dead tissue. It may be easiest to think of these as like inside-brain scars. Often they won't have any side effects unless they're pressing up against particular parts of the brain – in which case, you may need surgery to release the pressure.

Finally, there is a very low risk of radiotherapy causing a new brain tumour. After all radiotherapy damages all cells' DNA, so if it damages a healthy cell's DNA in such a way that it begins to multiply uncontrollably, then that could be the beginning of a new tumour. It may be the same kind or something entirely new to the tumour your radiotherapy was supposed to be getting rid of, and it could be benign, low grade or malignant. Thankfully the regular MRI scans you'll be having will pick up any new tumour at its very earliest stages. And the occurrence of radiotherapy-induced tumours is considered extremely rare.

Adjuvant treatment

This is a medical name for giving you two or more treatments at the same time, or each one directly after the other. The 'adjuvant' treatment is the one that backs up the main treatment. In most low grade gliomas this is exactly what will be recommended.

Again, the particular mix and match of adjuvant therapy will differ from person to person. Normally, you would expect surgery (if you can have it) followed by one or the other of radiotherapy or chemotherapy. That may then be followed up by the other one. In some cases, you may have radiotherapy and chemotherapy at the same time. In general, adjuvant treatments are considered more effective than single ones at both prolonging life and delaying malignant transformation.

There are loads of exceptions, based on genetics and tumour types, but it stands to reason that hitting your tumour hard with various different treatments at the same time, or in quick succession, is likely to offer better outcomes.

So how effective is treatment?

Here's where things get really complicated in brain tumours, because there are so many studies and each of those studies only analyse very small numbers and in each case deal with a very particular type of treatment and/or a very particular type of tumour. Saying all that, an overview does seem to indicate that the more treatment you have, and the earlier you have it, the better your prognosis. That's why it's called treatment.

What you'll be offered is likely to be that which the evidence suggests is most effective for your particular tumour, its subtype, its genetics, your age and other factors. By way of example only, and in order to avoid getting into too much detail, let's take oligodendrogliomas.

These respond particularly well to both radiotherapy and to chemotherapy. If the oligodendroglioma has some specific genetic strings missing (called 1P/19Q), which about 80% of them do, then their response to both treatments is particularly good. If they lack the deletion, the treatment is significantly less effective. At the same time, radiotherapy and chemotherapy for oligodendrogliomas – while generally proven to be effective at prolonging life and certainly effective at reducing symptoms – has not been shown to be more effective if given as soon as diagnosis has been made, compared with being given later on. However, earlier rather than later surgery *has* been shown to make a long-term difference.

Things are never simple are they? And even this relatively complex example is just to scratch the surface of the different types, subtypes and genetics, coupled with the different treatment regimes and even particular chemotherapy drugs and radiotherapy doses that have been proven, or not, to be more effective.

A half-day searching on Google about your tumour type and scientific studies on treatments is bound to turn up a few specific papers that offer a better picture. But note, many studies don't have a 'control' element. Surgeons can't, for example, randomly choose half of patients to undergo brain surgery and refuse surgery to others just because they're doing a study.

When searching for and reading scientific papers, there's a

chance of coming out more confused than when you started. But at least the papers might encourage searching and detailed questions of your medical team about what treatment they are recommending and why.

Consent

All this certainly doesn't mean we should always have treatment while we're still low grade, or even that our doctors will advise that we have treatment.

As with everything about brain tumours, the usual factors are at play: our age, the size of our tumours, growth rates, position, genetic makeup, ability to have surgery, our ability to deal with any side effects of treatment, and of course our own willingness to go ahead.

Doctors will take all of this into account before advising us, but here's the thing: it's still our choice. However much pressure you are under from doctors, family, others who've had brain tumours or the dreaded internet talk boards, at the end of the day it is you who decides to go ahead. And it is you who will sign the consent forms.

This book offers a tiny window on this stuff, but there's no replacement for asking questions of doctors and nurses, consulting brain tumour charities and the British Neuro-Oncology Society, getting other booklets, reading scientific papers and talking to other patients.

In April 2013 after a bout of intense and regular seizures, and after my neurologist discovered I had an abnormally high volume of blood vessels in my low grade glioma, he advised me to have the biopsy I describe above. He strongly suspected, he said, my glioma was transforming into a higher grade one.

The outcome of the biopsy was that I had an oligodendroglioma, but more interestingly the biopsy had *not* found any Grade III cells. On a microscope slide at least, I was still a low grade glioma patient.

Apparently my case was a matter of some debate among surgeons, my neurologist and others in my multi-disciplinary team: just because the biopsy hadn't recovered any Grade III cells didn't mean I definitely didn't have any in there. The needle may just have missed them. That, coupled with my seizures and the tumour's blood vessel growth, led my neurologist to advise I start treatment anyway. In other words, assume it was a Grade III oligodendroglioma and proceed from there.

This is where choice comes in: I decided I would prefer not to start treatment just yet. The summer holidays were approaching, which meant my children would be off school and I would be spending more time with them; my seizures had hugely abated since the biopsy; and, important to me at least, I was in very good shape for cycling.

Treatment was bound to come with some short-term, and possibly long-term, side effects. As long as it was a matter of treatment being a *maybe*, rather than a *definitely*, then I'd prefer to sit it out for another six months and see where we were then. I'd decided to strike a balance between my quality of life now and having treatment now. And I'd come down on the side of my good quality of life. If my health had not been so good, and if I'd not been able to spend decent time with my kids or ride my bike, I'm pretty sure I'd have gone the other way.

And guess what? When that six-month MRI did roll around, my neurologist reported that nothing at all had changed in my tumour during the summer. No growth, no increase in blood vascularity, no enhancement, nothing. I enjoyed the most wonderful summer with my kids, cycled some long rides and climbed some amazing mountains, and there had been no change. At the time of writing, that's exactly how things stand: I'm still living low grade and I've had no treatment for the tumour. Long may it continue.

> "We had put our faith in the doctors from day one,
> deferring to their qualified judgements and had no
> reason to change. The surgeon had reviewed my case
> and we were looking at when, and not if, the
> operation would take place. As soon as possible would
> have been my normal reaction. However, with the
> impending arrival of our daughter we wanted to get
> an idea of time scale. How urgent was the operation?
> How late could it be done without my health being
> put further at risk? The surgeon was very clear that
> delaying too long was not an option, while he
> understood our position. Six weeks post-birth was the
> outcome."
> *Duncan, 33, astrocytoma Grade II*

Why you can't simply do the sums

Wouldn't it be nice if doctors could add up the different
factors about our brain tumours: their specific type, size,
location and growth rate; then add those to our personal
characteristics like our genetics, age, health, diet and
metabolism; and then come out with a specifically tailored
treatment plan that is proven to extend our lives, prevent
transformation into a higher grade and generally make our
tumours less of a big deal?

Unfortunately, things are not that simple. The reason is
that low grade gliomas are relatively rare. There hasn't been
enough research, because there aren't enough patients, to
create a checklist of factors that ends up with the best possible
solution. And of course, everyone's tumour is different. As one
scientific paper states:

"The annual incidence of low grade glioma is about 4,700 cases per year [in the United States], which makes them one third as common as their higher grade counterparts. This relatively low incidence has prevented the development of standardized treatment protocols."[5]

Take my own case, for example. I have a low grade oligodendroglioma, that has specific genetic deletions, with a relatively high vascularity (blood uptake) score for my type of tumour. The tumour is located in the left temporal lobe, it is around 6cm at its longest point. I'm in my late 30s, am very fit and at the time of writing have not had radiotherapy or chemotherapy. All those factors added up together make me a very specific case. Your own factors make you another very specific case.

Since low grade gliomas are relatively rare anyway, how many trials of treatment pathways are there likely to have been that fit yours, or my, specific factors among people who have *also* taken part in a scientific trial? The answer is very few, if any. Certainly not enough to draw any concrete conclusions. The best we can hope for is wider generalisations, a broader classification based, say, on our tumour types and/or our genetics and/or our age. Anything else really casts the net into too shallow a pond to be useful.

No wonder doctors disagree about how low grade gliomas should be treated, and our consultants will only give us very general estimations of life expectancy and progress, if they're willing to offer anything at all. The data just isn't there.

Research trials

At any one time, there are dozens of research trials taking place across the UK on brain tumours. Unfortunately, according to The Brain Tumour Charity, only 3% of brain tumour patients are enrolled in one. A lot of this is simply down to not being asked to participate. Yet, the importance of research trials cannot be overemphasised: this is how developments in brain surgery, treatment and genetics happen.

But one thing does need to be made clear about research trials: very few of them are about experimental treatments. Some of us may be under the impression that research is all about testing a new serum that might give us a better chance of a cure. For the most part that's Hollywood blockbuster fodder. Instead, research trials are much more likely to be part of a long process of tweaking a certain type of treatment, or taking your brain cells and doing experiments on them, or trialling a new combination of drugs.

Individually, these trials might not make an enormous difference to your own condition. But added up with many other trials, they are slowly pushing forward diagnosis, treatment and may eventually lead to a cure for brain tumours more generally. It's worth noting that many of these trials are partly or even wholly funded by charities like The Brain Tumour Charity, Brain Tumour Research and Cancer Research UK. That's why support of these charities really does mean lives can be changed and saved.

There is a difference between research trials (likely to be developing understanding of brain tumours and their genetics) and clinical trials (which actually test treatments and other developments). At the time of writing, there are only a handful of research trials and no clinical trials including low grade gliomas in the UK and Europe. It's worth outlining them to offer an impression of the intricacies of what a research trial is really about. Though they may be out of date by the time you read this.

A study at Queen's Medical Centre in Nottingham is examining the family history of children and adolescents with low grade gliomas: how far are your family's genes likely to increase your risk of developing one? The National Brain Tumour Study is a UK wide project, involving up to a dozen hospitals, looking at the DNA of brain tumour patients of all kinds, including low grade gliomas.

University College London Hospital is investigating adolescent brain tumours, looking at their outcomes depending on which institution looks after their care. A study at the Institute of Child Health is examining developments in imaging of brain tumours. The Neuro-oncology Research Centre at the University of Wolverhampton is looking at genes involved in the development and treatment of a number of different tumour types. A number of hospitals are involved in a trial of a chemotherapy drug combination for treating low grade tumours that are growing back following treatment.

If you would like to be involved in a trial, you should discuss it with your medical team. If you're eligible, you'll be passed to the research team responsible. In many cases, simply a sliver of your tumour obtained in biopsy or surgery may be passed to the trial and you do nothing more. In some, your diagnosis alone will do and they'll test your blood, and perhaps that of your relatives, and will look at your DNA.

Only in a few cases might you be involved in experimental treatments, which may involve frequent trips to hospital, different drugs and side effects and likely more close monitoring by a medical team.

The latest UK brain tumour-related research and clinical trials are listed at The Brain Tumour Hub website and via the Cancer Research UK website. (See Resources)

Controversial and experimental treatments

Searches on the internet, and well-meaning suggestions by friends and family, may lead to consideration of 'experimental treatments', particularly abroad.

Often, these are legitimate clinical trials that are focused on trialling specific treatments or new discoveries. These are carried out according to all the usual medical norms like peer review, controlled trials and medical ethics. But very rarely would these legitimate trials be offering the possibility of a cure. They may only suggest a particular treatment may work better, or offer a better outcome.

Those trials and experimental treatments that offer a cure or offer a 98% chance your tumour will go away forever, particularly those you have to pay many thousands of pounds to be part of, often turn out to be very controversial indeed.

As a general rule, if it sounds too good to be true and is likely to cost you an awful lot of money, we should research and consult very carefully before pressing ahead. In particular, questions should be asked about whether the research or treatment is approved by local bodies governing medical trials, whether the trial has been peer reviewed in an established scientific journal and more generally whether the doctors and institutions behind it have received controversial or other media coverage.

Sadly, some families have paid inordinate amounts of money in the pursuit of hope, rather than a realistic chance of cure. I won't get here into the rights and wrongs of: 'You've got to try anything because it might just work.' Ultimately that's for patients to decide for themselves. I understand myself the desperation we all feel.

My personal approach is that if there really were cutting edge possibility-of-cure trials for low grade gliomas going on, they'd be going on among well known, respected brain surgeons, consultants and scientific researchers in the UK too. And I wouldn't have to pay for potentially life-saving treatment to be trialled on me.

7

Prognosis

THIS IS WHERE we get into deep territory. Depending on your point of view, you may wish to skip this chapter entirely.

If you *are* still reading, you're about to be disappointed. I know most of us want accurate statistics about our life expectancy and many of us spend hours looking for any indication of it, only to come away without any solid information. Unfortunately, that's the nature of brain tumours, particularly low grade gliomas. There are very few overviews or reviews of the scientific literature that can provide the solid answers we want. Where there have been scientific studies of prognosis, the literature offers only the outcomes for particular tumour types, which have undergone (or not) specific types of treatment, and which have (or don't have) specific genetic makeups.

It's not the aim of this book to assess all the scientific literature on low grade gliomas done over the last 20 years, and then to offer you an accurate, clean-looking table showing your life expectancy. And besides, low grade gliomas vary so much in their size, position, genetic makeup, and treatment developments are moving at such a fast pace, that any such information would be wildly inaccurate and certainly out-of-date the moment it was printed.

I'm no scientist. I freely admit to only being able to offer the same yet more woolly and sometimes contradictory answers. If that disappoints, at least I share the same frustration. That, again, is living low grade.

> "I saw little point trying to find conflicting data on the web which would probably only confuse me more. I'm very 'black and white' so the answers I was seeking probably don't exist."
> *Rory, 41, oligodendroglioma Grade II*

What follows is very much just a layperson's overview of what I have learned from my own research since becoming a low grade glioma patient in April 2012.

Information sources

I've used various sources, and not all of them agree with each other. They include: Cancer Research UK[6]; a great overview paper[7] on low grade gliomas published in 2011; another 2005 review[8] of nearly 1,000 glioma tumour patients in Zurich, Switzerland; the US website UpToDate.com, which aims to summarise current thinking and evidence on health topics 'to help healthcare practitioners make the best decisions at the point of care' and is written by peer-reviewed doctors; a similar site called MDGuidelines.com; and material from the American Brain Tumor Association.

These are very good places to start if you want to look into prognosis further, and there will also be specific information sources and scientific papers relevant to your particular tumour and treatment. But you should not take any of information in this chapter as a firm or conclusive prognosis. You should talk to your consultants about that because it will depend on your specific tumour type, any treatment you may have had or might have, and what other factors might affect your prognosis. Even then, your doctor might not be able to shed any brighter a light.

Need to know terms

Your *prognosis*, in basic terms, is what your life expectancy is with the particular type of tumour you have. Your *progression free prognosis* is basically the length of time your low grade glioma is not doing much: not growing significantly or transforming into a higher grade. That's after initial diagnosis, or after surgery.

Of course, there are loads of caveats, exceptions and outliers in any brain tumour prognosis. I'll cover these afterwards, because I'm guessing – if you're still reading – you'll want to get straight to the action.

There are two general ways that oncologists talk about life expectancy when they analyse statistics.

The *median*: This is the number of years when 50% of patients with that type of cancer have died. If there are 100 patients in a study and the median is seven years, then half of those patients died before the seven years and half afterwards.

A *specified time proportion*: Very different from the median and not to be confused with it. This is the proportion of patients who are expected to be alive after whatever time period is stated, say after five years. So if there are 100 patients and five years later 20 of those have died, then 80% of patients are still alive at the five-year period.

It's easy to see why the median and the specified time

proportion get confused, but understanding the difference between them is actually helpful. If you can get a median and a specified time proportion for your tumour type, then you'll have a clearer picture than only having one of them.

With the terminology more or less out of the way, here we go with our finger in the air statistics.

Gliomas in general

A pretty comprehensive scientific review of low grade gliomas summarised various studies, and concluded mainly that pinning down accurate prognosis for them is extremely difficult. Yeah, thanks for that!

The behaviour of low grade gliomas is highly variable and while some may remain stable for a long period, others differentiate sooner. Nevertheless the most recent data it cites gives a median survival rate for low grade gliomas of 'approaching 10 years'. This is stated as an improvement on earlier studies, but may be down to better imaging and earlier diagnosis than before. Younger patients, those with smaller tumours and those showing fewer disabilities down to the tumour tend to do better. Those who present with seizures also do better. Children tend to have a better prognosis, unless the child is very young indeed or the glioma is in a particularly dangerous place.

There are loads of other subcategories and influencers on survival. It's definitely worth reading Sally-Ann Price's excellent 2011 paper for more detail than I can provide here.[9]

Astrocytomas and mixed gliomas

Clinicians tend to group the two together, because the astrocytoma element of a mixed glioma is considered the more relevant one for treatment. But mixed patients do survive longer than pure astrocytoma patients.

According to a large European study, around 65% of

patients lived for at least five years and had no growth of tumour in that time. Astrocytomas transform into higher Grade III tumours, and when they do the statistics are not as good (27% living for at least five years). Grade IV astrocytomas have a worse prognosis still.

Another citation at MDGuidelines.com says 34% of astrocytoma low graders will be alive at five years if they don't have treatment, and 70% will be if they do. The Zurich review concluded a median survival rate of 5.6 years for low grade astrocytomas.

Oligodendrogliomas

These are very slow growing tumours and have a better prognosis than astrocytomas. About 66% to 78% live for at least five years, dropping to 30% to 38% living for five years when they are higher grade. The Zurich study found the median survival rate for low grade oligodendrogliomas was 11.6 years.

Ependymomas

Half of those diagnosed with an ependymoma will live for five years. Among children, 57% will live for at least five years with older children having a slightly better prognosis.

Meningiomas

Most meningiomas (90%) are low grade, and because they're on the outside of the brain most can be removed by surgery and shrunk by radiotherapy, effectively curing them. And 80% of people with a slow growing meningioma that hasn't been removed by surgery or radiotherapy will live for more than five years. So even if a slow growing meningioma cannot be completely removed, it may be controlled for a long time. Higher grade meningiomas are far more dangerous, with around 60% of patients living for more than five years.

Prognosis caveats

You may find the above statistics reassuring, or conversely you may find them scary. Either way, you're about to be thrown into more confusion. That's because statistics on life expectancy come with so many caveats. Once you've read them, you'll probably want to discard pretty much everything you've just read. Here we go, just to muddy the waters.

You're an individual, not a number

This is the most important thing to remember about prognosis. Statistics about death and life expectancy can only ever be based on groups of people and what happened to them, not on particular individuals and their particular cases. The smaller the group measured, the less reliable an indicator of life expectancy the study is likely to be. The most you can do is assume your own life expectancy lies somewhere on the graph. You can't presume or estimate where on the graph your own particular case lies. You have your own genetic makeup, your different tumour size, position, severity and any other number of factors. Just because someone else with your tumour and age died after five years doesn't mean you will.

Prognosis statistics are retrospective

By necessity, studies of prognosis can only look at what's happened in the past. Since the study finished, say 10 years ago, diagnosis, technology and treatment may have moved on enormously. Very often it does. That means you can't mirror a five-year-old study, which perhaps itself took five years to compete, on to what's happening right now. Chances are the numbers have changed, indeed probably improved, in the meantime.

The median isn't the middle

The median may well show that half of patients die after, say, seven years. But that doesn't mean 100% of patients will die by year 14. The median doesn't work that way. Stick with me because this gets a little complex.

Those who've survived more than seven years may, by the very nature of having already survived that long, be more likely to survive even longer. They may be the fitter patients, for example. The first 50% died relatively quickly as a group, compared to the second 50%, exactly because they weren't as fit. Many of those second 50%, due to their fitness, may be perfectly capable of living another 10 or 15 years after the first 50% have died. The median might be seven years, even though the last of the 100% died 30 years later. (Note: I'm not saying fitness is a always a prognostic factor in brain tumours. I'm using it as an example here.)

Conversely, this pattern can work in the opposite direction. Say a disease is degenerative: it gradually gets worse the longer your survive. By year seven, 50% have died. By year nine everyone else has died too. In this case, the median life expectancy is still seven years, even though we know the last of the 100% was dead by the end of year nine.

In other words, the median isn't the middle. It's the 50% mark, and that's not the same thing. The implication of all this is that you need to look at the full spread of survival rates, as well as the median, to get a more accurate picture of your chances. In fact, for some low grade glioma patients there are people who are still alive so many years after diagnosis, or who died from non-cancer factors related to old age, that their data means the median life expectancy simply has never been accurately determined. Where is the 50% survival point, when people in the study are still alive today? (A positive thought, if ever there was one.)

Where do we start, anyway?

This was the most difficult and frustrating aspect of prognosis for me to get my head around. And there are still far too many questions unanswered for me to get anything more than a finger in the air impression of my own prognosis, let alone tell you yours. The problem is this: when does the clock start ticking? Unless you start to drill down into very specific scientific papers about very specific tumours and very specific treatments, most prognosis information is very general indeed. Patients with a low grade tumour x have a median life expectancy of y, and that's all they tell you.

But does that life expectancy figure start from when the tumour was first discovered on an MRI? Does it start when the patient first noticed they were having headaches or seizures (sometimes years before they had the MRI)? Does it start when your consultant says: 'I think you have a low grade glioma?' Or does it start when you've had a biopsy that confirms you have a particular type of low grade glioma? And where does that leave those who've had an informal diagnosis, but not one confirmed by biopsy? Do they show up in the statistics or not?

And anyway. Do those general statistics include all low grade glioma patients lumped in together? Does it mean life expectancy as long as you have had all treatments available? Or does it mean your life expectancy if you don't have any treatment at all? The fewer of these questions answered, the fuzzier all the prognosis statistics become. And my experience has been that these questions are rarely answered, even in scientific studies, and the result is a very fuzzy picture indeed.

All of which is a long-winded way of saying: we just don't know, with any useful margin of accuracy, how long we're going to live. We don't know, with any useful margin of accuracy, what our progression free-prognosis is likely to be.

All we can really do is hope we come out at the better end

of the statistics, and note some of the prognostic factors (age, tumour size, genetics, symptom presentation) that have been generally agreed to confer a better survival rate.

I can't run around in a panic all the time, and I've concluded it's probably not best for me to retreat into a dark room and hide under the covers. Instead, I use the statistics to get a very basic impression of the lie of the land, then I concentrate on my quality of life and making the most of what I have got. Right now.

Looking for the right answers

It's human nature to be attracted towards positive news, and to avoid or discard information we don't want to hear. Welcome to the world of cancer, where this is multiplied 10-fold. My wife and I, even to this day, will Google brain tumours, low grade gliomas, or react to information about brain tumours in the newspapers. And then we'll cling to any positive information we can find.

Whether it be news of new treatments or changes in prognosis, we've recognised that when the news is good we pay it lots of attention. We research into it more, clinging to the little chinks of light it provides, no matter how poor the study, how hyped up it has been by newspapers, how experimental a treatment may be or even if it's a random comment on a talk board with no evidence behind it.

Meanwhile, when the news is bad or sad, we'll discard it: well, it's only a small study, it's not relevant to my situation, it isn't backed up by other evidence, it's only someone commenting on the radio. Looking at information in this way can be useful and it's entirely natural. Indeed, keeping on top of the latest news, opinion and other people's stories – whether good or bad – can be a way of dealing with our condition, as well as staying informed of latest developments.

But we've learned to take this kind of information with a pinch of salt. We acknowledge that leaning towards the positive and away from the negative is exactly what we're doing. Allowing ourselves to be bounced around by what we've found on the internet, or read in newspapers or worst on internet chatrooms, is only a small part of the wider picture. Try as we might, we know we won't be able to apply the same standards of criticism to the good news as we might the bad. But simply knowing that helps to put things in perspective, while allowing enough hope to filter through to keep us sane.

The end of low grade living

This is a book about living with a low grade brain tumour, not dying from one or from what a low grade may become in the future. There are some excellent resources for understanding what will happen if and when low grade brain tumours transform into higher grade ones (Grade III and IV), and the implications of untreatable or incurable brain cancer.

Suffice to say, for many of us there will come a point where we are no longer living low grade, the goalposts will move and our situation will change forever. In the meantime, low grade tumours are something we live with, rather than die from. Yet the fact that many low grade brain tumours often do, one way or another, end in a patient's eventual decline and death – however far into the future – cannot ultimately be ignored.

> "We have had to have very difficult conversations about care, death, all worst case but very realistic scenarios. As a cancer sufferer, coming to terms with eventualities is a necessity. But it is family and friends I feel will be more affected in the long run. These thoughts and discussions recur every few months

around the scans, making for a continuous cycle of
scan-result-wait."
Duncan, 33, astrocytoma Grade II

"I am very interested in my prognosis; I do a lot of
searching on the internet and discuss the situation
with my doctors at regular meetings. The doctors
were reluctant to give a life expectancy as there are so
many different variables that could affect the outcome.
The statistics showed that my life expectancy was
three to five years and this was confirmed in my
medical notes. That was three years ago and the MRI
scans show that my tumour hasn't changed size for
over a year now. So far so good! As far as dealing with
this, I think I'm philosophical. Apart from the
obvious, I keep fit and healthy and I am looked after
by my wife, who has more hassle by having to put up
with me."
Richard, 55, anaplastic astrocytoma Grade III

When first diagnosed, my wife and I ran around in circles
preparing for my death: there were things to do, arrangements
to be made, all in the fuzz of shock, grief and worry. I'd
started a detailed list of passwords and accounts for my bank,
my computers, my online accounts, just to make things easier
for my wife. I rushed around looking at my assets, and
deciding how to leave any I had to my wife and children. I
even started to think about songs for my memorial service.
And then, typical of my wife and I, we ran out of steam.

Things gradually didn't seem so urgent. We began taking
deeper breaths and began to prioritise. What really did need
to be done soon, and what could wait until later? Why spend
the life I do have left worrying about paperwork, instead of
getting on with living it? Some will of course find solace,

comfort and distraction in ploughing ahead with preparations and plans. Others will feel they don't want to 'jinx' their condition by planning for the worst, or simply can't bring themselves to contemplate it.

For us, we decided only a few things really did need to be done in the near future: our wills (after all, this is something we should have done anyway), an advanced decision (a kind of living will), and asking our closest friends and family about what their roles might be in relation to our children should it be necessary. Passwords and funerals? Well, they could wait.

Charities and hospices can provide information and support on terminal illness and the preparations that may need to be made. (See Resources)

8

Reasons to be cheerful

AT THE CURRENT time there is no known cure for low grade gliomas. Given time after surgery, most will come back. And eventually most are likely to turn malignant. But their very nature – that low grades tend to take a long time to do anything – means there may well be hope not only for patients in the future, but also for those of us living with low grade gliomas right now.

Recent years have seen a huge increase of breakthroughs in glioma research and treatment. Doctors and charities believe brain tumours may well be on the cusp of a tipping point: moving from a more or less hopeless case, to something that can be better controlled, better treated and – one day – perhaps cured.

A couple of decades ago, breast cancer was considered an almost incurable disease. Then, all of a sudden – and not least because there was a massive influx of funding for breast cancer research – the statistics started to get better. New surgical techniques were trialled and became common practice. New drug combinations were developed. New approaches to diagnosis and screening were used. Together they chipped away at breast cancer, taking the disease over the tipping point and radically changing the outlook for patients. Since the 1970s, there has been a steady increase in survival rates year-on-year. [10]

As talk among charities, consultants and researchers goes, brain tumours are just about where breast cancer was 10 to 15 years ago. Policy makers and researchers are coming to acknowledge that survival rates for *all* brain tumours are only the same now as the very worst cases of breast cancer. The statistics for brain tumours are only now starting to improve. Something more needs to be done. While to draw a direct parallel between breast cancer and brain cancer would be too far a leap to make, imagine if brain tumours got the funding, research and medical breakthroughs that breast cancer has enjoyed over the last 30 years?

Imagine if in the next 10 to 15 years, developments in research and treatment meant low grade gliomas could be controlled so well that they were almost as good as cured? That would mean many of us now living with low grade gliomas could see positive changes in our life expectancy *while* we're still very much alive. On particularly hopeful days, I can almost believe that, thanks to developments in treating the disease, I might just live long enough for my brain tumour never to catch up with me.

So, what are these exciting developments in brain tumour research? They boil down to better understanding of how brain tumours work (their genetics), getting better at removing more of them (surgery) and getting better at seeing them in the brain so diagnosis can be made more accurately and more tailored treatment offered (imaging).

I outline here just a few exciting developments in what's

going on in all kinds of treatments, but they're just the tip of an increasingly large iceberg. I hope they give an impression of what is already possible, and what might be possible in the future.

Developments in surgery

The most promising development in surgery techniques for low grade gliomas is what has become known as the 'pink drink'. It's something scientists are trialling right now across the world and are having some significant success with.

One of the key problems about brain tumour surgery is that you need to remove as much as possible to make a significant difference to both the quality of life and the life expectancy of patients. And if you can remove tumour cells but not the healthy tissues around them, you're less likely to damage parts of the brain that make the body work. As Dr Colin Watts, consultant neurosurgeon at the University of Cambridge, who is at the forefront of this research put it:

> "In certain areas of the brain, such as those
> controlling movement, a millimetre can make the
> difference between a patient being disabled, or being
> able to walk out of hospital."[11]

Add to this that tumour cells don't often look much different to healthy brain tissue and that some cells are bound to remain if they're lurking in and around creases in the brain, and you can see how complex brain surgery becomes. This is where the pink drink comes in, because it can make brain tumours glow. That's right. Glow!

The pink drink (called 5-ALA and which isn't actually pink) can make brain tumour cells appear a glowing pink under ultraviolet light. That means a brain surgeon, armed with an ultraviolet torch, can distinguish better between the tumour and the healthy brain tissue around it.

So more brain tumour can be taken out. Surgeons can also see bits of tumour lurking in nooks in the brain they wouldn't otherwise have seen. And they can avoid cutting away bits of the brain that aren't glowing.

The science is very new, but the implications are encouraging. While concentrating right now on high grade tumours, if the technique is rolled out more generally the news for low graders might be good too. Those low graders who previously wouldn't be considered for extensive brain surgery may soon be able to have it. And those who do have it may come out of surgery in a better state than before.

If you can stomach it, there are some amazing videos of the pink drink in action during brain surgery on YouTube.[12]

The importance of genetics

Genetics has to be the most exciting, interesting and hopeful aspect of all research into treatment and cure of low grade gliomas. Simply put, if scientists can understand what's going wrong with the DNA of low grade glioma cells and identify the shared characteristics of those developing low grade gliomas, then there really is hope for the future. And I'm not just talking the distant future.

I'm talking real progress in targeted chemotherapy and radiotherapy treatments that could help currently diagnosed low grade patients – that means you and me – to live longer. As the 11th Annual Frye-Halloran Brain Tumor Symposium 2012 at Massachusetts General Hospital put it, there is no less than a 'molecular revolution' taking place right now in low grade glioma genetic research. And as the report of the symposium put it:

"Understanding the role these genetic alterations play in brain cancer initiation and progression will help lead to the development of novel treatment modalities than can be personalised to each patient, thereby helping transform this now often-fatal malignancy into a chronic or even curable disease."[13]

Remember, this is very much a layperson's book not a science one. With that in mind, here's my best attempt at tackling brain tumour genetic research and its implications.

Every cell in your body, including tumour cells, have at their very heart strings of chemicals called DNA, and these in turn are split into genes. What's important is that genes are masses of information that control how cells grow, react and generally go about their business. If a particular part of a gene gets mixed up or mutated, that's obviously going to mean the cell doesn't grow or react how it is supposed to.

These mutations are given technical names like IDH1 and ATRX. We don't have to know or care what they mean. We just need to know that low grade gliomas tend to have some of the same mutations or the same presence of particular genes. Understanding this genetic makeup of tumours might help prevention, or at least assist in delaying transformation to higher grade tumours.

For example, scientists have identified that where some genes have particular mutations, then particular treatments like radiotherapy and chemotherapy work better than if the tumour doesn't have those errors. All in all, it's extremely complex but extremely important. And that's why, if you have a biopsy or surgery, it's very likely that you'll have a test for the genetics of your tumour. Doctors already know enough to allow your own particular tumour's genetics to determine the treatment they offer you. And that possibility has only been around for about 10 years. Imagine the potential of another

10 years of research into this stuff?

The science is not clear cut. The presence or absence of particular genetics in tumours doesn't seem to be enough by itself. The really complex part scientists are looking into is the role played when tumours have a particular *combination* of mutations and presences of particular genes. The role played by these combinations seems to be more important than a single gene marker by itself.

By way of example, here are just a few highlights of what's known:

IDH1

In this case, mutation is good! This mutation is found in a majority of low grade gliomas (and obviously higher grade ones that have transformed from low grades). It is an exciting new discovery and has been cited as 'perhaps the single most prominent prognostic factor for overall survival after [the grade of the tumour]'.[14] Already, it is understood that the presence of the IDH1 mutation means certain types of chemotherapy work better. But scientists are also looking at the effectiveness of taking more of the tumour out depending on the presence or not of the mutation.

1P and 19Q

Where these particular genes are missing in oligodendrogliomas, patients live longer. Plus, tumours respond better to radiotherapy and particular types of chemotherapy. So obviously identifying the loss of these genes can help doctors to diagnose the tumour, as well as plan treatment.

ATRX

News for astrocytomas patients here, if you have this genetic alteration. Those with it, as well as the IDH1 mutation, do significantly better than those with IDH1 alone. One of the key ideas behind identifying ATRX alterations seems to be that they form part of a 'signature' of astrocytomas. That means better diagnosis, and therefore more tailored treatment.

Combinations of genes

Scientists are finding that oligodendrogliomas that have (1) lost the 1P and 19Q genes; and (2) do have the IDH1 mutation, also tend to have (3) a mutatation in a gene called CIC. Meanwhile oligodendrogliomas and astrocytomas without this combination of (1) and (2) were rarely found to have (3). The biology is showing that the relationships of all three of these genetic markers seem to be involved somehow in these types of tumours, rather than one gene acting by itself. Unlocking the relationship between genes like this could offer a massive clue for developing treatment and understanding brain tumours in the future.

What is gene tailored treatment?

I am criminally simplifying here, but the way genetic strings – or mutated ones for that matter – go about their work might be part of what makes brain cancer happen and progress. If chemotherapy drugs can be developed to block the mechanism that they make happen, then somehow cancer can be delayed or stopped in its tracks.

Multiply all this up across the different genetic markers in brain tumours, and you end up with very specific tailored treatment that blocks very specific mechanisms caused by these genes. The more pathways blocked, the science is hypothesising, the stronger the resistance to the cancer. As one presentation at the 2012 conference on brain tumour genetics concluded:

"Carefully designed clinical trials using drug
combinations may offer the key to developing
successful cancer treatments."[15]

If you're up for some serious medical jargon, with more
than a few incredible extra insights into low grade glioma
tumour genetics, how they work and how they're driving
treatment, I strongly suggest taking a look at the whole
conference proceedings. There's even a podcast to listen to.[16]

Better imaging of brain tumours

Another battle ground for the better tackling of all brain
tumours, including low grade ones, is improving the imaging
of them. If doctors can see more of the tumour or particular
characteristics of the tumour on a computer screen, after
MRIs or other imaging techniques, then the better and more
specific their prescribed treatment is likely to be.

A problem with gliomas is that they infiltrate into the rest
of the brain. They don't stay put like one spherical lump. As
one consultant complained:

"There is an understanding that the degree of
invasion differs with individual tumours, and yet they
are all treated the same."[17]

So getting a clearer picture of the tumour and where its
tentacles reach out into the brain, will give doctors and
surgeons a clearer idea of its size, its rate of growth and any
other characteristics. Take for example, radiotherapy. A better
image of the brain tumour means radiotherapy can be
targeted more specifically, and less of the surrounding tissue
will be damaged. So that's why development of better brain
imaging is important. But what is going on in this field?

Already, radiographers can track the pathway of blood through the brain by effectively 'dyeing' the blood so that it is picked up by an MRI scanner. On the computer screen, the blood vessels in and around a tumour can be seen. Imagine if a dye could be produced that chemically stains a particular protein that is wrongly produced by one of these gene mutations.

Then an MRI or other form of imaging might be able to 'see' these proteins, thereby creating a better picture of the brain tumour (which has the stained protein) compared with the bits of the brain that don't have the stained protein. All of which means better estimations can be made about what kind of low grade brain tumour it is, even without doing a biopsy (some brain tumours produce some kinds of proteins, some produce others), as well as allowing closer monitoring of tumour size, diffusion into the brain and position.

Research into this kind of 'staining' for mutations and other genetic markers is moving at pace, in line with a better understanding of brain tumour genetics. Once again, it puts brain tumour genetics at the heart of research into future treatment.

Even without genetics, improvements and new discoveries in brain imaging techniques are set to make a difference to how the disease is monitored and treated. Conventional MRI scanning only goes so far, giving an impression – but rarely a very accurate picture – of the invasion of glioma tumours. Tumour cells have been found up to 2.5cm away from where conventional MRI scanning has identified them.

Newer techniques are looking at the very biological makeup of tumours and how they infuse into the brain to improve their imaging. Low grade gliomas, for example, tend to grow along tracts of white matter in the brain. Imaging techniques like Diffusion Tensor Imaging (DTI) can show up where tracts of white matter are being pushed out of the way by a growing low grade glioma, thereby showing their extent and size. Over a period of time, mapping of the movement of white matter can show the growth and infiltration of the tumour. One study found that the less disrupted the white matter around the tumour, the better the patient's life expectancy.

A final word

THE SAD TRUTH is that many with a low grade glioma tumour will one day die from the condition. That may not be in the next few years, or even in the near future at all, but a low grade diagnosis does mean many of us are more likely to die from our tumours than from something else.

Yet the very longevity of this type of tumour does offer an undeniable glimmer of hope that things may change; a real hope that death from most types of low grade gliomas may not be inevitable in the future. While my wife and I retain a philosophical and resigned outlook – we do know my brain tumour is very likely to end my life – I cannot deny that we both can also see a chink of light in the future.

With my particular tumour, the median life expectancy from diagnosis appears to be a full 14 years. There's every chance I could live that long or many years longer. It's a long time and 14 years is just the median.

With science and better understanding of our particular type of brain tumour, the prospects are ever improving. When you consider the rapid pace of cancer research, treatments, drugs and knowledge, there is a chance that in the next decade or so things will have changed so much that death from brain tumours becomes much rarer. Or at least, those all important median life expectancies become longer and longer. There's every reason to believe that brain tumour research and treatment really is right now at a tipping point.

This isn't to instil false hope. Every low grader needs to understand our condition well enough to know the difference between what is possible and what is probable. Yet it would be untrue to say that given the pace of progress in the field that low grade tumours will always carry the same prognosis they currently do.

Once the Cinderella of cancers, brain tumour research is now receiving more funding than ever before. New discoveries about brain cancer, how and why it develops, and what might help to prevent or treat it are being made all the time.

It seems that living low grade is partly all about managing our own hope: striking that delicate balance between the chance of change in the future, and being realistic about how quickly those changes may come about.

Some can only think in a hopeful way, putting all of their emotional investment in the belief that change will come in time for them. Indeed, for some this may be the only way they can regard their condition. Others will try to avoid this kind of hope, preferring to err on the negative side, perhaps allowing themselves to be pleasantly surprised if developments are more positive.

Every low grade tumour patient will have to find their own level. But at least for all of us, the subjects of future prognosis and treatments are far from clear cut. Things in medicine do change, achievements are being made. Once fatal diseases have been and still are being cured, or at least kept at bay for longer.

In other conditions, little progress has been made in decades. I guess we'll never know until it happens. Until then,

I hope understanding of low grade gliomas develops, including how they work and how they affect patients' lives.

First, that we have a possibly life-limiting disease, and that's enough in itself. Second, that we have a constantly changing, ebbing and peaking range of symptoms and side effects, as well as emotional responses, that we, our family and our friends have to deal with on a weekly, if not daily basis. But third, there can also be long periods of time when nothing much is happening, and that we sometimes wonder what all the fuss is about.

Embracing this trinity, and getting medical practitioners to understand the complexity of our lives, is what I and many others have found living low grade is really all about.

*

I hope you like the way I write and have been interested in my story. I publish a regular blog about living with a brain tumour. You can be first to hear when I post new blogs by signing up at www.bicyclesandbraintumours.co.uk

I love to hear from my readers. Please do connect with me on Twitter (@gideonburrows) or via www.facebook.com/LivingLowGrade

No pressure, but it would be fantastic if you could review this book on Amazon, Goodreads or any other review site you use. If you've found it helpful and think others could benefit too, please do tell people via your social media and other networks.

Thanks so much for reading!

Gideon Burrows

Resources

100 Questions and Answers about Brain Tumors
Virginia Stark-Vance, Mary Louise Dubay (Jones & Bartlett, 1993)

The Emperor of All Maladies: A biography of cancer
Siddhartha Mukherjee (Fourth Estate, 2011)

Like a Hole in the Head: Living with a brain tumour
Ivan Noble (BBC Books, 2005)

Living with a Brain Tumour: A guide to taking control of your treatment
Peter Black (Holt Paperbacks, 2006)

Low Grade Gliomas
Sally-Ann Price, Stephen Price et al. (Advances in Clinical Neuroscience and Rehabilitation, March/April 2011)

The Median Isn't the Message
Stephen J Gould (Discover, 1985)

Molecular Genetics of Low Grade Gliomas: genomic
alterations guiding diagnosis and therapeutic intervention
(*The 11th Annual Frye-Halloran Brain Tumor Symposium, 2012*)
http://thejns.org/toc/foc/34/2

Why Millions Survive Cancer
Lauren Pecorino (Oxford University Press, 2011)

*

Astrofund
Astro Brain Tumour Fund focuses purely on low grade brain
tumours, raising funds for research and support projects,
sharing information and raising awareness of the challenges
of living with a low grade brain tumour.
www.astrofund.org.uk

brainstrust
A UK-based brain cancer charity, dedicated to improving
clinical care for brain tumour sufferers and providing co-
ordinated support in their search for treatment. Provides
support and advice at the point of diagnosis and beyond, as
well as information on treatment and care.
www.brainstrust.org.uk

The Brain Tumour Charity
The UK's largest dedicated brain tumour charity, committed
to fighting brain tumours on all fronts. Funds scientific and
clinical research into brain tumours and offers support and
information to those affected, while raising awareness and
influencing policy. Its aim is to improve understanding,
diagnosis and treatment of brain tumours.
www.thebraintumourcharity.org

Brain Tumour Hub

Created by brainstrust, this aims to be a comprehensive and authoritative database of the brain tumour support resources and UK-based brain tumour clinical trials.
www.braintumourhub.org.uk

Brain Tumour Research

Campaigning charity and umbrella group of smaller charities which concentrates on fundraising, lobbying and raising awareness. Funds brain tumour research at UK hospitals.
www.braintumourresearch.org

British Neuro-Oncology Society

Formal group of clinicians promoting research and education in all aspects of brain cancer.
www.bnos.org.uk

Cancer Research UK

Funds over half of the UK's cancer research and considered the country's leading expert charity on all kinds of cancer. Also provides information, support and cancer awareness.
www.cancerresearchuk.org

Cancer Research UK research trials database

Searchable database of many current cancer-related clinical and research trials in the UK, including brain tumours.
www.cancerresearchuk.org/cancer-help/trials/

Macmillan Cancer Support

Concentrates on providing support and information on cancer in the UK, as well as advice and information on every aspect of the disease. Also funds Clinical Nurse Specialists and other medical and therapeutic staff across the UK.
www.macmillan.org.uk

Acknowledgements

This book wouldn't have happened without the time, openness and generosity of the dozens of low grade and other brain tumour patients who were willing to share their story. Thank you. I have been moved, impressed, astonished and humbled in equal measure. Ultimately, this is your book.

Thanks too to Louise Taylor and Kate Kershaw at The Brain Tumour Charity, and Helen Bulbeck at brainstrust for their interest in and support for the project, particularly for putting me in touch with patients. Thanks to my wife Sarah Mole for her thorough critique of my writing. It is always welcome and always creates a far better book in the end. Thanks to my good friend and colleague Jennifer Campbell for her excellent proofreading. Acknowledgements also to the information team at The Brain Tumour Charity for fact checking and correcting. Any remaining errors are mine.

Thanks to my own medical team. Particularly my neurologist and my two CNSs. I ought to be more grateful to you and the NHS for everything you've done for me and thousands of other brain tumour patients.

Notes

[1] Epilepsy Action has an extremely detailed outline of the rules at https://www.epilepsy.org.uk/info/driving/driving-licences-group-1-rules#group1 (Accessed 30 October 2014)

[2] MRI scans may be done by a less qualified *radiographer*, while analysis of the scans and delivery of radiotherapy is always done by a *radiologist*

[3] MRI scans are often done by a less qualified *radiographer*, while analysis of the scans is done by a *radiologist*

[4] The main sources for the information in both the Treatment and Prognosis chapters are P. Black (2006) *Living with a Brain Tumor*, Holt Paperbacks; Macmillan Cancer Support (2010) *Understanding Brain Tumours*; V.Stark-Vance (2011) *100 Questions and Answers about Brain Tumors*; and Cancer Research UK *http://www.cancerresearchuk.org/cancer-help/type/brain-tumour/* (Accessed 9 October 2013)

[5] D. Rotariu et al. (2010), *Malignant Transformation of Low Grade Gliomas into Glioblastoma: a series of 10 cases and review of the literature*, Romanian Neurosurgery

[6] Cancer Research UK, http://www.cancerresearchuk.org/cancer-help/type/brain-tumour/treatment/statistics-and-outlook-for-brain-tumours (Accessed 5 September 2013)

[7] S.Price et al. (March/April 2011), *Low-grade Gliomas*, ACNR, volume 11, number 1

[8] H. Ohgaki, P.Kleihues (June 2005), *Population-based Studies on Incidence, Survival rates, and Genetic alterations in Astrocytic and Oligodendroglial Gliomas*, Journal of Neuropathology and Experimental Neurology, volume 64, number 6

[9] S.Price et al. (March/April 2011), *Low-grade Gliomas*, ACNR, volume 11,

number 1

[10] Cancer Research UK, *http://www.cancerresearchuk.org/cancer-info/cancerstats/types/breast/survival/breast-cancer-survival-statistics* (Accessed 9 October 2013)

[11] Lecture to The Brain Tumour Charity audience by Dr Colin Watts, 21 March 2013

[12] YouTube, *http://www.youtube.com/watch?v=3IQsLkbrU_U* (Accessed 10 September 2012)

[13] P.S.Jones et al. (2012), *Molecular Genetics of Low Grade Gliomas: genomic alterations guiding diagnosis and therapeutic intervention. 11th Annual Frye-Halloran Brain Tumor Symposium,* Neurosurgery Focus

[14] Lecture to The Brain Tumour Charity audience by Dr Colin Watts, 21 March 2013

[15] P.S.Jones et al. (2012), *Molecular Genetics of Low Grade Gliomas: genomic alterations guiding diagnosis and therapeutic intervention. 11th Annual Frye-Halloran Brain Tumor Symposium,* Neurosurgery Focus

[16] Journal of Neurosurgery, *http://thejns.org/toc/foc/34/2* (Accessed 10 September 2013)

[17] S.J.Price et al. (December 2011), *Imaging Biomarkers of Brain Tumour Margin and Tumour Invasion,* British Journal of Radiology

Printed in Great Britain
by Amazon